PAIN IS NOT WHAT IT SEEMS

ADVANCE PRAISE

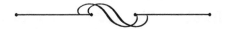

"Dr. Anita Hickey possesses the wisdom and talent to present a challenging subject in a language that all can understand. The book is a road map for transcending an out dated paradigm on how society and medicine views pain and suffering. Furthermore, it explains what the individual can do to transform their life. Richard Cecil said, "Eloquence is vehement simplicity." This quote epitomizes her work. The book is a must have and gift for all."

Kathleen J. McDonald
D.O., MA

As an expert in the field of Pain Medicine, Dr. Anita Hickey powerfully addresses how to treat pain and not just "manage" it. A much needed and well-researched book for patients and physicians. It is perfectly titled and will change the way you think about pain. Pain is not what is seems, and this incredible book will tell you why."

Alane B. Costanzo, M.D.-Pain Medicine

"Dr. Hickey shares her extensive experience in treating chronic pain as both a personal journey of professional expansion and as an academic gathering of research and treatment modalities. Throughout her book she describes for the lay public the newer understandings we have about the underlying causes of chronic pain. More importantly, she connects different modalities that can lead someone with chronic pain, not to eliminating pain, but to an expanded sense of an empowered self, able to create a more satisfying, self-defined life."

Thomas M. Fitzgerald MD
Medical Director, Southlake Psychiatry PC, Davidson, NC
ABPN Board Certified General and Addiction Psychiatry

"Dr. Hickey's book, *Pain is Not What it Seems* has assisted me in discovering that I am in large part responsible for creating my own health through thinking, feeling, food, exercise and meditation. This book should have been called, *You are Not Your MRI*. I now understand that while a laboratory test, x-ray or MRI is a snapshot - static and unchanging. We are living beings and can change the ongoing processes in our bodies and mind. The power is in our own mind, feeling and higher self. Dr. Hickey has a keen intellect and has compiled a treasure trove of research on the subject of pain and the treatment of pain, both from the allopathic and complementary and alternative medicine perspectives. Her book gives us the scientific understanding of why it is critical that we take back responsibility for our own health, using the medical system as a valued recourse and partner while putting our health and well-being back where it belongs, squarely in our own hands."

Vera Auge, BSN

"Theologian C.S. Lewis said, "Pain is God's megaphone to rouse a deaf world." In her book, Dr. Hickey addresses holistic healing on all dimensional levels not just one isolated, physical component. Her presentation is in a manner that is easy to understand! It's plain

English & not a medical school text book; an absolute must-read for all desiring a truly therapeutic, restorative lifestyle!"

Tanya Ponder, CRNA
CAPT (ret) U. S.

PAIN
IS NOT
WHAT IT
SEEMS

*The Guide to
Understanding and Healing from
Chronic Pain and Suffering*

Anita Hunt Hickey M.D.

NEW YORK

LONDON • NASHVILLE • MELBOURNE • VANCOUVER

PAIN IS NOT WHAT IT SEEMS

The Guide to Understanding and Healing from Chronic Pain and Suffering

© 2019 Anita Hunt Hickey M.D.

Published in New York, New York, by Morgan James Publishing in partnership with Difference Press. Morgan James is a trademark of Morgan James, LLC.
www.MorganJamesPublishing.com

ISBN 9781642793000 paperback
ISBN 9781642793017 eBook
ISBN: 9781642793611 audiobook
Library of Congress Control Number: 2018911692

Cover Design by:
Chris Treccani
www.3dogcreative.net

Interior Design by:
Christopher Kirk
www.GFSstudio.com

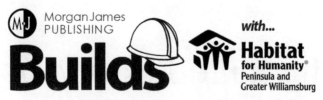

Morgan James is a proud partner of Habitat for Humanity Peninsula and Greater Williamsburg. Partners in building since 2006.

Get involved today! Visit
MorganJamesPublishing.com/giving-back

To my precious children, Alicia Macknight, Sarah Elizabeth, and Ethan Patrick, and my granddaughter Una.

TABLE OF CONTENTS

INTRODUCTION

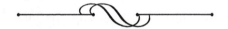

*"We must all die. But if I can save him from
days of torture, that is what I feel is my great and
ever new privilege. Pain is a more terrible lord of
mankind than even death itself."*
– Physician and philosopher Albert Schweitzer 1875 – 1965

I could always take pain – physical pain. My mother
said that even as a baby, I never cried when she took
me to our family physician to get my shots. I grew
up as the fifth of seven children. My parents grew up
during the Depression, my father in Salina, Utah and
my mother in Santa Barbara D'Oeste, Brazil as a third-
generation descendent of American immigrants to
Brazil. My father was a veteran of WWII, a University
Professor and my mother a linguist. They were strong
and determined, "pull yourself up by your bootstraps"
individuals. It was church every Sunday and sometimes
during the week, wake up early on weekends to pull
weeds, wash windows, clean the house, help with baking

the bread or with taking care of the many creatures (dogs, cats, monkeys, horses, and other animals), which we acquired throughout the years of my childhood and adolescence. If it wasn't work, we were shaken awake in the still-dark morning, then driven by my father to the top of one of the many canyons or to the mountains near our home in Flagstaff, Arizona.

By the time I was eleven, I had climbed down and up Havasu canyon, a branch of the Grand Canyon which is still inhabited by the Havasupai Indians, thirty-three times. I knew the canyon's trails, river, and waterfalls nearly as well as our home. When I was in high school, my parents left Phoenix and the Thunderbird Graduate Institute for International Studies (where my father was Academic Dean and Dean of Students and my mother a foreign language instructor) to live and work with the Havasupai Indians and so the canyon truly did become our home. Pain, physical pain, was the inseparable consequence of the long hikes, long runs, and horseback rides through the forests and occasionally getting thrown off of a horse. The rewards were many and outweighed the pain (at least in retrospect). I remember swimming in the blue green waters of Havasu Canyon, the immense silence and beauty of standing on the canyon ridge or at the top of Mt. Agassiz, the inexplicable bond between horse and human after the long rides. Making it uphill on the climbs was always the challenge. Arriving at the top or going downhill seemed a reward in itself.

It was the emotional pain that I could not take. The pain of someone crying, the pain of cruelty, of lack of compassion or feeling for others. I became known as the mediator in our family, the peacemaker, though I think now that this was possibly more in an effort to alleviate my own discomfort than as a grand gesture. Retreating into reading, schoolwork, and the woods and nature were my other childhood escapes. And so, it seems somehow fitting that I would choose the medical fields of anesthesiology and pain management as my professions. Both gave me the ability to take away the pain of others. As an anesthesiologist, there is the "magic cocktail" that we give to the patient as we prepare to leave the preoperative "holding area." This instantly dulls the emotional pain of anxiety, fear, anger, and sadness. Depending on the surgery to be performed, once arriving in the operating room, an injection to numb the nerves and remove all ability to feel any pain, or a "general anesthetic" is administered to take away all sense of time passing while the surgeon uses his or her consummate skills to remove, repair, or replace an offending part. Then there is the waking up. Emergence from anesthesia is rather like a child being woken from a deep sleep by his parent. The patient is then taken to a recovery area where nurses, like kind aunts or uncles, attend every need, bringing warm blankets and injections from Morpheus to ward off the pain. The patient wakes to a white dressing or cast over the incision as the only record of the Delphic revision that has occurred. Then, as a parting gift, the bottle of "pain" pills to last until the healing is complete. Ah, and then every chronic pain patient likely knows the stern look of the surgeon or pain physician that accompanies the request for a second bottle of opioids, as if the agreement has somehow been broken. "Why do you still have pain," the look seems to say, "when my other, 'good' patients, are grateful and doing well?" Physicians in the past have often succumbed to the easy temptation to comply with the patient's request as this is the easiest way to end the visit and see the next patient on time by giving the patient what they "want" rather than going through a painful and often prolonged discussion of the dangers and ineffectiveness of opioids for the treatment of chronic pain. With the tens of thousands of deaths from the opioid crises in just the last year, the pressure is on physicians to rely less on the prescription for more opioids and more on less-lethal non-opioid alternatives. The patient, they know, will not take no for an answer easily. For the patient, the promise of relief seems to have been broken and the opioids are a less desirable but at least reliable escape from the constant, intolerable pain. They somehow will escape the fate of the tens of thousands. They will be "smarter" and will find a way to stop the pain and get off the pills.

Whether your chronic pain started after injury, surgery, cancer, or "wear and tear" from work, exercise, or sports, this book is for you. It is for you if you continue to have chronic pain that may have even worsened after surgery, medications, physical therapy, chiropractic therapy, injections, and even acupuncture, massage therapy, and other complementary and alternative treatments including diet and exercise approaches. If you can't live with chronic pain any longer, this book will help you understand why you are where you are, how to finally stop covering up the pain, and how to treat the underlying cause of your pain.

In my role as a pain management physician, I am often asked if the epidural or radiofrequency ablation is a "band aid." I tell them that yes, whether it is medication, a procedure, or a surgery, everything that we do for patients is a "band aid," but that there are things that can be done to treat the underlying cause of their pain.

After decades of studying both Eastern philosophy and medicine in addition to conventional Western medicine, then delving deep into the science behind pain and healing (which is not taught in medical school or even in most residents or fellowship programs), I have learned how to translate the science of how to heal from pain into practical steps that many of my patients have used successfully over the years to gain hope where previously there was only despair. I have included references in this book from masters of healing from Eastern medicine as well as from pioneer physicians and scientists from conventional Western medical approaches whose techniques can be used by those with chronic pain. Their books and writing may not have been written to address chronic pain, and thus may have been overlooked as a resource for patients with chronic pain.

I was urged to write this book by many of my patients, who felt empowered to finally take back their lives and begin their own individual journeys to healing after learning of the many simple, scientifically proven solutions to reversing chronic physical and emotional pain and chronic disease.

This book is not a substitution for medical care or advice from your physician. In writing this book, I do not intend to dissuade the reader from obtaining medical advice or care when it is recommended or indicated, but rather to learn evidence-based approaches and an understanding of how both the underlying causes of chronic pain, and simple methods for healing, can be utilized in your everyday life to vastly improve your ability to reverse chronic pain and disease.

"Why haven't I heard about this before?" my patients and colleagues ask. I tell them, "Because our current health system is built to manage illness, not to treat the underlying cause of disease." Although there is currently a movement among health organizations and physicians in the United States to utilize a preventive, integrative, and holistic approach, they must frequently rely on "membership fees," cash payment, grants, or philanthropic gifts to cover the costs of complementary and alternative treatments and educational approaches that are not covered under our current health system.

Many patients, physicians and other healthcare providers and administrators are not familiar with the definition of "Integrative and Holistic Medicine" and how it differs from the conventional Western approach to medical treatment. Integrative medicine is not the same as complementary and alternative medicine. It combines approaches from both Western and complementary medicine that have the best scientific evidence or merit. A holistic approach is one that looks at the individual as a whole person, seeing them as more than a physical body to be "fixed," more than a "head case" to be medicated. A holistic approach sees how our mind, body, emotions, occupation, background and culture, social circumstances, and spiritual beliefs all affect our health. It looks to help the patient find the underlying causes of disease and works with the patient to find treatments, and to motivate the patient, in keeping with the patient's beliefs and desires. An example of this approach can be found at the Salt Lake City Veteran's Hospital, where the integrative medicine program includes American Indian healing traditions, acupuncture, yoga, and other healing mind body approaches. The VA is a leader in this approach and on its website describes this new way of approaching medical care:

"VA facilities are shifting from a health care system focused primarily on treating disease to one rooted in forming continuous healing relationships and partnerships that support Veterans in achieving their greatest overall well-being. The result is a whole health approach, which is a bold redesign of health care focused on empowering and equipping Veterans to take charge of their health and well-being. Guided by a personalized health plan, VA's Whole Health System considers the physical, mental, emotional, spiritual, and environmental elements that work together to provide the best quality of life for each Veteran. As we reconnect with what matters most in our lives and learn new approaches to help us live life to the fullest, VA health teams will be there each step of the way. THIS is the VA of the future … The Pathway is a partnership with peers where Veterans are empowered to explore their mission, aspiration, and purpose, and begin their overarching personal health plan." (1)

As the VA suggests above, the current billing codes, insurance coverage, payment systems, and appointment times are designed for the treatment and management of disease symptoms, not for treating the underlying cause of disease or for educating patients on how to prevent chronic pain and disease. For this reason, individuals in the U.S. paid $34 billion out of pocket in 2007 for complementary and alternative approaches to health and well-being for treatment modalities not covered by insurance plans.

Dr. David Eisenberg reported in his landmark article published in the Journal of the American Medical Association that in 1997, visits to complementary and alternative practitioners exceeded visits to primary care physicians by more than 243 million. He reported that consumers disclosed that they were looking for natural therapies, healthy diets, and information regarding the benefit of nutrition, exercise, and stress reduction strategies to prevent disease, while focusing less on the diagnosis and treatment of the symptoms of chronic disease. (2)

For this reason, I believe that educating physicians and administrators of hospitals and health plans is not enough to change our current paradigm (which is based on the scientific principles of the 1400s to the 1700s during the era of the scientific revolution) to one which reflects the holistic principles of a systems approach to healing, one which is based on the more recent Nobel prize winning science of the 1800s to the present (again, not taught in medical schools).

The path to healing for each of us must be as unique as our face, our life history, and our fingerprints. This is why we must ultimately travel our own journey into healing. My hope is that this book and the references herein of many dedicated researchers, physicians, and healers will serve to provide general guidelines that have been shown to be successful and effective for many patients suffering from chronic pain and disease with easy to apply instructions on how to utilize and adapt these tools in your unique life.

In part one (chapters 1, 2, and 3), you will learn the importance of transitioning from a limited to an unlimited mindset as you come to understand that developing a new way of thinking is essential for healing. I will introduce you to scientists who have unlocked the secrets of the vast healing capacity of human beings, utilizing the untapped intelligence of the human being. You will also be introduced to simple techniques that have been shown to change the biochemistry affecting inflammation, the immune system, and the hormonal or endocrine system within minutes in measurable ways; techniques which change the brain as seen on advanced imaging studies and change the function of our genes in just weeks; and techniques which show reversal instead of progression of chronic disease on computerized tomography as measured by advanced imaging over time. You will develop a deep understanding of why our emotions and beliefs are immensely more powerful tools for healing and reversing the underlying cause of pain than any procedure or medication.

In part two of this book (chapters 4, 5 and 6), I will help you to understand why it is essential that you create your own optimal environment and connections in order to improve your ability to heal; how to create and maintain positive life choices while being true to yourself; how to create your own "Blue Zone" to increase your longevity and the quality of your life; and what living in the present moment has to do with healing from pain. Chapter 6 alone can change your pain and transform your life.

Chapter 7 will help you understand what specialty doctors, such as neurosurgeons and orthopedic surgeons, pain physicians and interventional neuroradiologists know – that your pain may or may not be related to findings seen on your standard imaging studies (magnetic resonance imaging (MRI), x-rays, computerized tomography). You will come to understand the processes that cause pain, which cannot be seen on imaging studies. Also, you will learn how and why images can improve over time, not just get worse.

Finally, in chapter 8, you will understand that it's not only what you eat that predicts your health and ability to heal, you will understand the significance of the latest research on diet and epigenetics (changes in our DNA or genes that occur in response to our thoughts, emotions, exercise, etc.) in regard to healing from pain, and how certain foods as well as how much and when you eat can promote healing and reverse biologic aging and pain.

At the conclusion of this book, it is my aspiration that you will have renewed hope and understanding of the unlimited resources both within yourself and available to you for little to no cost. You may have already seen improvements in sleep, mood, pain level, relationships, and overall well-being. You will also understand that you, as a health consumer, have greater power than physicians, healthcare organizations, corporations, and politicians to change the way that we treat pain and disease in our country. You as a health care consumer can choose options which include natural therapies, information regarding the benefit of nutrition, exercise and stress reduction strategies to prevent disease. You can choose less focus on the diagnosis and management of just the symptoms of chronic disease and ask our system to address the underlying cause of chronic pain and disease. Using American ingenuity, I believe that we can create an economic model that recaptures the lost productivity of the discouraged, burnt out, and disabled and halts the burgeoning rise of costs associated with the treatment of preventable chronic pain and disease. I believe that we can create an economic model which prevents the tens of thousands of annual deaths associated with reliance on opioids for the relief of pain and suffering.

PART ONE

Chapter 1

CHANGING THE PARADIGM

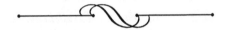

*"Parts are seen to be in immediate connection, in
which their dynamical relationships depend, in an
irreducible way, on the state of the whole system
(and indeed, on that of broader systems in which
they are contained, extending ultimately and in
principle to the entire universe). Thus, one is led to
a new notion of unbroken wholeness which denies
the classical idea of analyzability of the world into
separately independently existing parts."*
– Physicist David Bohm

I think we only see the beginning of a thing or
a journey when we look back, in recollection.
During my fourth year of undergraduate study as a
chemistry major and biology minor at Northern Arizona
University, I signed up for the senior honor's class titled,
"Mapping Reality." I was president of the physics club,
and excited that the course requirements included texts
by renowned physicists covering topics ranging from

quantum mechanics and subatomic particle physics to cosmology. Since my first love was literature, philosophy, and history, I was also curious to study the comparisons drawn to similarities between the wisdom of ancient sages, Eastern philosophy, and Christian mystics to the understanding of reality according to the Nobel-winning scientists of the 19th and 20th centuries.

The course included books such as, *The Tao of Physics: An Exploration of the Parallels between Modern Physics and Eastern Mysticism* by Fritjof Capra; *The Dancing Wu Li Masters: An Overview of the New Physics* by Gary Zukav; *Taking the Quantum Leap: The New Physics for Non-Scientists* by Fred Alan Wolf; *Time Space and Medicine* by pioneer mind-body physician Larry Dossey, MD; and Eastern philosophy books, such as *The Three Pillars of Zen* by Roshi Phillip Kapleau. The concepts revealed in this course and in these books were very profound and changed my worldview. For example, we think of the map of the river as being the same as the river, forgetting that the map is not the river, teeming with life and in a state of constant change due to the many forces that shape its course and path. The map does not have the smells and feel and sounds of the river and does not teach us what the river does when we go to its banks or travel down its course. All of us unconsciously accept the map of our life that we are given. We are taught that we are children, grow up, and become old and sick and then die. This is what the map is. That then is what must happen to us. This is what we were taught, and this is what we know. My parents had heart disease, back pain, cancer, and died in pain. I will also have heart disease, back pain, cancer, and will die in pain. That is the map, and thus reality.

The new physics and the ancient sages both arrived at the startling realization that the map is not reality; that mind, body, and spirit are one, intrinsically, inarguably, just as matter and energy are one. Each thing, each being, is unique. Mind and spirit can affect the body and the body can affect the mind and spirit, and most radically of all, everything and everyone is not separate. Everything and everyone is connected, so each one of us affects the whole, the web, the ocean of reality.

After completing my undergraduate studies, I attended medical school at the University of Arizona in Tucson where two courses in particular added to my understanding of this emerging paradigm change within science and medicine. One of our professors was renowned mind-body pioneer Dr. Andrew Weil who introduced us to the concept of integrative medicine. A human being is more than just a body yet is not an unembodied mind or a spirit. A human being is an inexplicable fusion of mind, body, emotion, environment, community and spiritual aspect. The aspect of spirit is often mistaken as being synonymous with religion. Although our religious practices and beliefs can shape our spiritual practices, we can think of the spiritual aspect of being as that which gives us courage, integrity, commitment, compassion, meaning and the will to move forward to fulfill our commitments and our lives.

Integrative medicine is a patient-centered holistic approach to healing, taking into account all aspects of the human being (mind, body, and spirit), including lifestyle and environment, which affect overall health and well-being. Dr. Weil taught us that an integrative medicine approach utilizes conventional Western medicine and complementary and alternative medicine approaches that have been shown by high level research to be safe and effective. It is a holistic, patient centered approach, which empowers the patient to take an active role in their own health and well-being.

While emphasizing the strengths and value of conventional Western medicine, which saves countless lives in cases of acute illness such as strokes, heart attacks, trauma, and infections, he conceded that conventional Western medicine has not been as effective in treating many chronic illnesses due to a model which emphasizes treatment and management of the *symptoms* of chronic disease, without addressing the underlying *causes* of the disease itself. He said frankly that, as physicians, whether we agreed with them or not, studies showed that our patients would seek complementary and alternative treatments which address their desire to improve their underlying health with exercise, healthy diets and supplements, spiritual guidance, and stress management strategies. We could either bury our heads in the sand (and then, our patients would just not come to us for guidance regarding these approaches), or we could become educated as to the best evidence for the various complementary therapies and treatment modalities. We could then help guide our patients to seek those therapies that could be of the most benefit to them, with the least risk for harm.

During the next two years, Dr. Weil introduced us to complementary medicine practitioners and modalities ranging from ancient Chinese and Japanese healing methods such as acupuncture, Hara diagnosis and therapy, and Jin Shin Jyutsu, to more modern alternative treatment modalities, such as Craniosacral therapy and Kinesiology, then to traditional healers such as Curanderos, Indian medicine men, and even a fire-walker. He also revealed case histories of patients, which divulged the amazing capacity for healing as well as the frighteningly powerful potential for creating illness and disease that we as human beings possess. I would learn more later of the amazing effects of our own thoughts and emotions from the research of Candace Pert, PhD, who had, just a few years earlier in 1979, discovered the opioid receptor at John Hopkins University and who would go on to discover the astounding origin of emotions, and the reason that emotions were so powerful at creating and healing human disease.

In my final year of medical school, in 1987, I enrolled in an elective course entitled, "Medical Ignorance." The two physicians who taught the course were a surgeon and an internal medicine physician who had both studied under the famous author, poet, essayist, educator, and researcher Lewis Thomas, MD ("Lives of a Cell"), while he was professor and chairman of the Department of Medicine at NYU-Bellevue Medical Center. They had been greatly influenced by this remarkable physician. At the end of the course, each medical student received a "Doctorate in Medical Ignorance." Although "medical ignorance" might seem quite contrary to the goal of becoming a physician, I soon understood, that in order to pursue knowledge, one needed to have a "beginner's mind" much like a practitioner of Zen Buddhism. As such, those who are most learned and wise, know how much more there is to learn.

In our current medical system, the doctor is often looked up to as one whose knowledge and recommendations are set in stone, much like the ten commandments – the ultimate authority – and that what is published in the medical journals and texts is "fact." We were introduced to the strange but true concept that there is an inverse relationship between the amount published on a subject and what is understood or "known" about that subject. An example of this is smallpox (of which very little could be found in medical journals or books since its eradication following the development of the smallpox vaccine), versus the Acquired Immune Deficiency Syndrome, or AIDS. This was 1987. There were volumes upon volumes of research journals, theories, conference proceedings and abstracts on AIDS, yet the cause and nature of the disease was a mystery in the 1980s and no conventional medical treatments had been discovered. The tenets of medical ignorance were: "When you read the medical literature, don't read to memorize the 'facts,'" but ask yourself, "what questions are being asked?" "What do we still not know?" and "How can we discover the answers to those questions which are being asked?" After this experience, I came to the essential understanding that while medical understanding and knowledge was in a highly fluid and expansive state, the practice of medicine is less so and does not always reflect what we know. This is due in great part to the social and economic structure and organization of healthcare, where change is tempered by tradition, economic and political forces, and the fear and distrust of change itself.

During my second year of medical school, I applied and was accepted to a United States Navy Health Scholarship program. While many of my classmates did not understand why I joined the service, I felt a strong devotion to serving our country and caring for our courageous service men and women, their families, and our veterans, due to our father's service in World War II and my older brother's service in Vietnam as a combat corpsman for the United States Marines.

My older brother had been seriously injured while in Vietnam, received two purple hearts, and was treated over the course of six months at Naval Medical Center San Diego. He then applied and was accepted to an enlisted to officer program during which he received both his undergraduate and medical education. He returned to Naval Medical Center San Diego as a Lieutenant with eleven years of service in 1979. After his internship, he was trained as a flight surgeon and served for three years in the VXE6 Squadron, which supports the research teams in the Antarctic. He then returned to Naval Medical Center San Diego for residency training as an anesthesiologist. After reading his letters from the Antarctic, in addition to my altruistic motivations, I yearned for the adventures and unique opportunities available to military physicians.

The next several years of my life were filled with the rigors, discipline, exhaustion, and excitement of medical training. After successfully completing a transitional internship and residency in Anesthesiology at Naval Medical Center San Diego with focused training in complex obstetrical anesthesia, I enjoyed many leadership opportunities as an anesthesiologist and Naval Officer at Naval Hospital Camp Pendleton, Naval Hospital Naples Italy, Naval Health Clinic New England, Naval Medical Center San Diego, deployments to the Subic Bay in the Philippines, Guantanamo Bay in Cuba, Australia, aboard aircraft carriers in the Gulf, and aboard both the USNS Mercy and USNS Comfort Hospital Ships.

Pain management training is a requirement during our residency training, and I had gravitated toward it, both during residency training and in my subsequent duty stations as I felt great gratification relieving the suffering of patients with relentless pain and enjoyed the technical aspects of treating patients with advanced injection and infusion techniques.

When I transferred to Newport Rhode Island, I resolved that I would seek focused fellowship training in pain management. I found that many of my patients had pain that I could easily treat with such simple techniques as trigger point injections for areas of persistent painful muscle spasm and epidural steroid injections for neck or back pain radiating to the arms or legs due to degenerative disc disease, causing inflammation and associated irritation of spinal nerves.

I remember one patient, a retired Air Force Colonel, who came in with great difficulty walking due to extreme pain radiating down his left hip, thigh, and leg with numbness and tingling of his left foot and toes. His L5-S1 disc (the disc between the fifth lumbar and first sacral vertebral bodies) had herniated and a piece of the extruded disc had become separated from the rest of the disc and was resting on the nerve root, which supplied the now excruciatingly painful part of his left leg. He was taking Ibuprofen multiple times daily.

I took his lumbar MRI films next door to consult with my orthopedic spine surgeon colleague. Since the patient did not have any "red flags" such as loss of control of his bowel or bladder or any significant leg weakness, he agreed that a conservative trial of epidural steroid injection was much less of a risk for the 78-year-old retired Colonel than spine surgery. I performed the epidural steroid injection and when the Colonel returned two weeks later, he stated that he had gone from using pain medication daily prior to the epidural steroid injection, to perhaps one pill every week. He returned two weeks later and said that not only was he not using any Ibuprofen at all, but that coming in for follow ups was interfering with his busy life. He thereafter would just leave a note with our administrative assistant now and then: "Just returned from New York sailing with the New York Yacht Club, doing well. Don't need another epidural yet!" Two years later, he returned for a second epidural steroid injection, from a colleague who had taken my place after my transfer to my next duty station

Some patients were not so easy. Their pain was widespread, not easily treated with medications, and not alleviated with even the most technically perfect injections. Their pain was often in multiple locations and accompanied by anxiety, depression, insomnia, migraine, and digestive disorders. It was at this time that I was the "fly on the wall" to a conversation that changed my practice. Two of the nurses from the operating room were talking in the lunchroom. I overheard one say: "Last year I had severe neck pain and pain radiating down my left arm. I went to the spine surgeons and they told me that I needed a cervical fusion. I'm too young for a fusion! I paid out of pocket to go to one of the doctors of acupuncture here on the island and after a few treatments, all of my neck and arm pain was gone." The other nurse then said: "That happened to me too! About two years ago I was in a car accident. I had back pain, muscle spasms, and neck pain. The doctor sent me to physical therapy and gave me non-steroidal anti-inflammatory drugs and muscle relaxants. A year later, I was still going to physical therapy, taking non-steroidal anti-inflammatory drugs and muscle relaxants. Since my insurance doesn't cover acupuncture either, I paid out of pocket for acupuncture and about six treatments later, I didn't have any neck pain, back pain or muscle spasms." After eavesdropping on this conversation, I made a commitment to complete rigorous training to obtain certification in medical acupuncture.

When visiting my older brother, who had retired from the military and was in a full-time pain management practice, I was asked by the owner and lead pain physician to join the practice. She was excited to have me offer medical acupuncture to their patients, in addition to the conventional pain management techniques that were being offered. Two of the other physicians in the practice were doctors of osteopathy and were utilizing craniosacral and osteopathic manipulation techniques in addition to usual medication and injection techniques. The practice also had a psychologist who taught patients about how their thoughts and emotions could affect their pain.

I decided to delay my fellowship training, leave active duty service for the Navy Reserve, and join the pain management practice. Utilizing acupuncture, I was able to holistically address all aspects of the human being and address depression and anxiety along with multiple areas of pain. However, although I had great success using acupuncture on patients where no other conventional treatment had been successful, I was now to begin my education in the "real" world of medicine.

In the military there was no need for the complexity of medical billing. All of our patients had coverage through the military health care system so we treated the patient according to best medical practice and did not worry about whether the procedure would be "covered" by the patient's insurance plan. I did not realize that all medical billing codes are developed and approved by a panel of physicians from the National Medical Specialty Societies, insurance companies, and the American Hospital Association, and approved by the American Medical Society Board of Trustees. If there is not a code for it, you cannot bill for it.

As a civilian pain physician, I was discouraged from utilizing acupuncture too frequently due to the poor reimbursement of this modality as compared to the conventional interventional pain procedures.

Additionally, many of the insurance plans did not cover acupuncture and "cash out of pocket" for acupuncture was not an option for most of our patients, who were either hard-working middle-class individuals, on worker's compensation, retired and on social security and Medicare, or on social security disability.

The practice overhead for medical practice is high due to the many legal, credentialing, governmental and organizational requirements, rent, coding staff, billing staff, and nursing staff. When physician payments are cut by Congress, in order to continue to meet expenses, practices must see more patients in less time, and holistic interviewing and treatment takes more time and pays less than conventional medical approaches, even when it is covered by insurance plans or cash out of pocket payment. I was thus encouraged to treat patients with pharmacologic and conventional interventional approaches, which had much higher monetary reimbursements.

After two years in private practice, I returned to active duty. I had missed serving the military and retired military population and their family members. I missed the intangible benefits and opportunities of being a military officer. I also realized that I would be much more likely to be able to utilize acupuncture and other holistic and integrative approaches in the military health care system. This is so, as the military leadership supports a preventive approach which emphasizes healthy lifestyle choices, self-reliance, and resiliency, all of which a holistic patient centered approach to medical care fosters.

I found myself in the upcoming years working with many military and civilian physicians looking to change the model of medical care from one of the patient as passive recipient of health care, to that of an active participant in his or her own well-being. Many physicians had become tired of just treating symptoms and wanted to shift the medical paradigm of one where instead of just being "providers of medical care" we could provide options for preventive approaches and health and wellness education in order to empower patients to develop healthy lifestyle choices and improved overall well-being.

It was several years until I was able to apply for, and be accepted to, my pain management fellowship. I had to apply and be accepted by the military selection process and then by the Pain Fellowship Program at Harvard's prestigious Beth Israel Deaconess Arnold-Warfield Pain Management Center and Boston's Children's Pain Treatment Center. Both centers are practice and research leaders in utilizing an integrative multidisciplinary approach, utilizing the best evidence of conventional medicine and interventional pain treatment, together with the most effective psychological, rehabilitation and complementary approaches to not only relieve pain, but to empower patients to reach a state of well-being.

Not Healing

What took me by surprise was that many of our patients were still not getting better with mindfulness classes, yoga, Tai Chi, Qigong, nutritional, and mobility education! After taking a hard look at my own lifestyle, which mirrored that of my patients, I realized why. We are all over-doers! As Americans, our ancestors did not stay by the fireplace in the old country. They travelled mountains and oceans to come to a new land where they could pull themselves up by their bootstraps to achieve the American dream. My military patients were even higher on the scale of over-doers, risk takers, high achievers. The lifestyle is work hard, play hard, sleep little. "Pain is weakness leaving the body." And if there has been stress, trauma, even horror or abuse, then "be strong," "stuff it" in a box somewhere, and get on with life. Like me, most Americans think, "I can use the yoga, Tai Chi, Qigong, and meditation training to get back to the high tempo game, but once I feel better, after the injection, after the massage, after the yoga, it is high speed again with no more time for lollygagging around." It was then that I realized that, in order to truly heal, we had to understand the underlying cause of chronic pain, what it truly takes to heal from chronic pain and disease, and what we have to do to maintain a life of health and well-being.

Meditation: "Experience of Unbroken Wholeness"

Sit in a quiet place where you will not be disturbed in a comfortable chair, back supported, shoulders and arms relaxed, legs uncrossed, and feet flat on the floor about hip width apart.

Close your eyes and relax your breathing. Focus on your breath, how it feels as it enters your nose and lungs, as your belly naturally expands with the in breath and relaxes with the out breath. Let your breathing be effortless.

Now, starting at the top of your head and slowly scanning down the body to your feet and toes, as you come to any areas of tension, allow the tension to melt as if from ice, to water, to vapor and then to space.

Feel the relaxed connectedness of all of your body, thoughts, emotions, and the part of you that is awareness and consciousness. If worries or "to do" thoughts arise, let them drift away like a cloud and return to the awareness of your breath.

Now sense the space around your body. Sense the unbroken wholeness and connectedness. Allow all tension to dissolve. Remain in this state of deepening relaxation for 36 inhalations and exhalations. Before resuming your normal activities, slowly open your eyes and look around. Remember that you can return to this feeling of relaxation, well-being, and connectedness at any time.

Chapter 2

DEVELOPING AN
"UNLIMITED" MIND SET

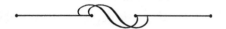

Step one: See New Possibilities. Frontiers of Medicine and Science

> *"We cannot solve our problems with the same thinking we used when we created them."*
> – Albert Einstein

Understanding the Physiology of Healing

Through extensive study of the nervous system during my pain fellowship and subsequent research into the use of the Stellate Ganglion Block for the treatment of Post-Traumatic Stress Syndrome. I began to realize, as I came to understand the way that pain is processed in the nervous system, that nonscientists (and indeed most physicians), have very little understanding of the complex systems in the body that can both create chronic pain and help us to heal from chronic pain.

Through years of intense study of research involving these systems, I came to understand how certain simple techniques work to heal pain. The problem was that patients did not understand *why* they were being taught techniques, such as meditation and yoga. They did not understand why they were being given these tools. They thought that the techniques were to help them relax, to not feel stressed out, and to feel good about themselves so that they would not be depressed or suicidal.

Since we have very a very limited time frame for patient appointments, it took a few years before I was able to find a way to explain to my patients, within a few minutes, the true purpose of pain; how acute pain (such as a stubbed toe) is much different than chronic pain, why and how chronic pain develops, and why only they can heal from chronic pain … no one else can do it for them or to them, why everything that we do for them (such as medications, injections and even surgery) will not treat the underlying cause of their pain.

First of all, I start out by telling them the astounding truth that while most of us look at pain as the enemy (certainly the patient who suffers from intractable pain does), pain is truly our best friend. When I say this, their eyes open wide! "How can pain be our friend?" "Well," I say, "the reason that your pain is so very hard to treat, is that pain is processed in many different pathways and centers in the brain in a very complex way, because, without pain, we would not survive. Without pain, we would die. Pain is there to protect us. Pain is our means of survival, both as a species, and as an individual. Human life exists and persists only within certain limits of temperature, pressure, acidity, alkalinity, strain and stress."

Acute pain tells us when something is outside of the limits compatible with health and life. It tells us when something is too hot, too cold, too sharp, too heavy, and when something is going to threaten our survival. Those children who are born with the rare genetic disease that prevents them from sensing pain do not live very long, as they cannot sense when their environment is too hot or too cold and cannot regulate body temperature. They cannot tell when something is too sharp and so are injured, get infections, and die.

Patients with diabetes and those with other neuropathies that impair the ability to sense pain, often injure themselves, acquire infections, and need amputations. Even those of us who can sense pain often ignore the messages that pain gives us. We just take the pain pills and continue to do what we think we have to do, day after day, until the message becomes so loud that we can no longer ignore it. Then we feel betrayed by the pain. We give up and think that, "it has won" and that we can no longer live the life that we had planned or the dreams that we had dreamt.

The Difference between Acute and Chronic Pain

Most people, even most physicians who are not pain specialists, do not understand that just like a computer, there is a hardware and a software component to pain. First of all, a hundred people can have the same injury, surgery or accident, and not all of them, not even most of them, will develop chronic pain. Most will completely heal. It has been shown however, that the change from acute to chronic pain can occur in just 8 to 16 hours of large scale or persistent pain signals being sent to the spinal cord and the brain.

In those who develop chronic pain, the software of the body's nervous system changes how and where pain is processed. This makes chronic pain much more difficult to treat than acute pain. Chronic pain is defined as pain that persists past the period where we would normally expect the body to heal after an injury, a surgery, or an illness.

According to the International Association of Pain, pain is "An unpleasant sensory and emotional experience associated with actual or potential tissue damage or described in terms of such damage." (1) The current standard teaching about chronic pain is that it no longer serves a purpose as a warning that we are at risk for actual or potential tissue damage. Although this is true, just as acute pain is a warning to protect us from danger or harm that might threaten our lives, chronic pain is just as important a warning. It tells us that the underlying systems of our body (the immune system, neurohormonal system, and autonomic nervous system) are out of balance and thus we are not able to heal.

In Eastern medicine and philosophy, it is taught that disease manifests initially on the energetic level (emotional, mental, and spiritual levels) of the individual. If it is not halted or not treated at this stage, it travels deeper to the functional level (creates pain, stiffness, movement, and function difficulties). If it is not diagnosed and treated at the functional level, it may travel deeper to the level of the organ and present as a more severe disease. For example, the bladder meridian or channel runs from the inner eye region, over the head, down the sides of the spine, the back of the legs to the outer heel and fifth toe. Disharmony at the energetic level might manifest as depression, fear, or lack of motivation. At the functional level, it could manifest as back or neck pain, and at the level of the organ it could manifest as recurrent bladder infections, or even bladder cancer. An acupuncturist or Eastern medicine physician thus strives to diagnose and treat a disease at the earliest possible stage- meaning at the energetic level or at the latest when it presents at the functional level, as the longer the disharmony persists, the harder it is to treat.

Acupuncture, Jin Shin Jyutsu, Healing Touch, Reiki, meditation, Qigong, Tai Chi and other complementary and alternative healing arts have their action in harmonizing the underlying systems of the body (immune, neuroendocrine, autonomic nervous system) (2) and this is why they are able to help with so many different types of health conditions. In this sense then, chronic pain is also a valuable warning and friend which, if we heed its admonitions and take the necessary steps to help our body heal, may help us prevent more severe disease in months or years to come.

How do acute and chronic pain differ? First of all, because pain plays such an important role in our survival, the processing of pain is very complex and involves the immune, sensory, hormonal, and inflammatory systems, both in the periphery of the body and in the spinal cord and brain. When tissue injuries occur, inflammation occurs both from the injured tissue and from the response of our own immune system. The inflammatory chemicals are transmitted to the spinal cord and brain and can result in an increased state of inflammation throughout the entire body. We also have ways of down regulating or turning down this inflammatory state. These down regulating influences include our "endogenous" or internal, self-produced opioid system and mental and emotional states such as distraction and self-efficacy or self-regulation (I'll talk about this more later as this is very important in preventing chronic pain).

Our pain "matrix" is made up of multiple centers in the brain which all interact to create our individual response to pain. The "first order matrix" is made of brain centers that process our initial response to a painful event. The "second order matrix" is made of centers in the brain that mirror our individual response to and interpretation of the painful event.

Depending on our response or interpretation of the pain, we can either turn pain down or turn it up. Because of this, pain experts and researchers stated recently that, "Transition of acute to chronic pain may be minimized by early recognition of risk factors and early biopsychosocial pain management." (3) This is because pain involves not only the sensation of pain, but also the emotional component of suffering. Thus, emotional distress, stress, anxiety, depression, and pain can co-activate each other in a patient who has been wired for chronic pain.

It is important to note that, just as this software change toward chronic pain can occur in just a few hours, it can also be *re-wired* or *reprogrammed* in the opposite direction in a short period of time. One example of this in acute pain is the use of virtual reality and distraction on burn units. Even with pain medications, pain can be excruciating for these individuals. Using distraction and Virtual Reality, these patients noted very significant decreases in their pain during burn dressing changes. (4)

The Typical American Lifestyle

In order to understand how to change the programming of chronic pain, we need to understand the effects of the typical Western lifestyle on our chronic pain and chronic disease. This is good news. By understanding the cause of chronic pain and how to reverse chronic pain, we are also coming to understand and treat the underlying cause of chronic disease.

How can this be? We all know about the "fight or flight" adrenalin-run part of our nervous system. It is the caffeine driven, work twelve-to-fourteen-hour day system that we rely on in our modern day to achieve the American Dream lifestyle. We wake up in the morning, drink coffee to wake up, then more coffee to keep going, come home and sit down in front of the television to "come down" from the nonstop engine of our day, then take a drink or a pill so we can sleep (if we even can sleep). The next morning, not having really slept well, we drag ourselves out of bed for the early morning commute, drink more coffee, and then do this day after day, year after year until we finally "break down." We spend our life "working out" and "training" our "fight or flight" nervous system, which is only supposed to be used for emergencies. In the typical American and Western global industrial lifestyle however, every day is one emergency after another. We are continually running on "fight or flight mode" without knowing that this is our "break down" mode and that the body also has a "rest, relax and repair" mode that we can use to rebuild our bodies. What? Why did we not learn about this?

So, yes, there are two nervous systems in the body. Our "fight or flight" system is only a small part of the overall picture. There is the somatic nervous system, which supplies our muscles, and the nerves, which transmit non-painful sensation. Then there is the autonomic nervous system, which supplies all of our internal organs such as the heart, lungs, kidneys, bladder, spleen, intestines, our blood vessels, our skin (including sweat glands and the capillary system which help us to regulate or maintain a temperature compatible with life). It also supplies feedback and information from and to our sense organs (eyes, ears, nose, taste) and our skin (which is the largest sense organ).

The autonomic nervous system is divided into two parts: the sympathetic nervous system, which we know as the fight or flight or adrenalin part of the nervous system, and the parasympathetic nervous system. The pain fibers or nerves are associated with the sympathetic nervous system. So, when we have chronic pain and chronic stress, these co-activate one another. What we don't realize is that the sympathetic nervous system is the breakdown mode. If we stay in this mode day after day, year after year, the body continues to break down. Think of a company or a ship that is operating day after day, week after week, and month after month in a full out emergency mode. Soon the personnel and the equipment would break down, unless time was taken for sleep, relaxation, and restoration of personnel and equipment.

The "rest, relax, and rebuild" mode is the parasympathetic nervous system. The parasympathetic nervous system helps us to properly digest, absorb, and eliminate our food, helps to decrease our heart rate and blood pressure after periods of stress, helps us to obtain restful restorative sleep, dilates vessels to supply our tissues with nutrients, oxygen, and growth factors needed to replace injured cells and tissue with new.

When we activate the parasympathetic nervous system, we are in the rebuild and restore mode. The parasympathetic nervous system is in relationship with the other underlying systems of our body such as the immune system and the neuroendocrine or hormonal system, which act together as a "super system." By training the parasympathetic nervous system and bringing it into balance with the sympathetic nervous system, we can bring the other systems of the body into harmony, balance or a state of "coherence" and reverse the imbalances at the root of chronic disease and chronic pain! But how do we do this? (5)

The problem is that in modern society, no one tells or teaches us how to activate or train the rest, relax, and rebuild mode. All of the activities we take on, even exercises and diet, are to enable us to continue to fuel more of a frantic daily rat race like the "give 200%" model or the "burn out, then retire and spend your time going to the doctor" American lifestyle. We were told that methods such as meditation, Qigong, and yoga, can help with stress, but we don't have time to "take a break" every day to deal with stress. No one told us that these are like "going to the gym" or "training" the parasympathetic nervous system. Just like going to the gym once a week, once a month, or once a year will not build a muscle, doing yoga, meditation, or Qigong once a week or month will not adequately train the parasympathetic nervous system to repair and rebuild our bodies, our minds, and the spiritual aspect of our being.

One More Piece of the Puzzle

I'm sure that most of you have heard of stem cells and stem cell therapy. Most of us think that in order to utilize the amazing ability of stem cells to help with regeneration of the body we have to pay out of pocket (since these therapies are not covered by insurance policies) and have someone inject "stem cells" or "platelet-rich plasma" or other stem cell attracting substances into the body. However, scientists have found that even old, sick patients produce their own stem cells, not just throughout the body, but even in the brain!

When we are young (in stem cell language that means when we are under twenty-five years old), our stem cell proliferation rate or ability to replace old worn out or injured cells, is about 83%. Between the ages of twenty-five and thirty-five, there is a dramatic decline in our stem cell proliferation. That is why in our mid- thirties, we often start having problems with weight gain, even while eating "the same things we always have," not healing quite as well after injuries, etc. Fertility also has been shown to decrease by this age in most people. By age sixty, if we live the average American lifestyle, our stem cell proliferation is only about 10%!! What recent research has also shown, however, is that we can increase stem cell proliferation, even in old age, with certain foods, moderate exercise, and mindfulness techniques. I hope you are starting to see a trend here. My study of the ancient science of Ayurvedic medicine helped me to understand at an even deeper level why mindfulness may be the most important of the three (diet, moderate exercise, and mindfulness), if we are to heal from chronic pain and disease (more on this in chapter 8).

Step 2: Even You and I Can Do This

I think that knowing what we are capable of as human beings, even as novices in the activities which promote healing, gives us hope that even we can do this and hope is critical to the process of healing. My patients find it incredible that recent advanced imaging and electroencephalogram studies (graph of brain waves representing electrical activity in the brain) show that in just eight weeks of daily meditation or yogic breathing for an average of twenty minutes daily in NOVICE meditators, the prefrontal cortex of the brain (the part of the brain which we use to make executive decisions), measurably increases in thickness. The studies also showed an increase in communication between the two sides of the brain and whole brain coherence (communication between the various centers of the brain). (6)

In long-term meditators, these changes are even more profound. That is why elite athletes and multimillion-dollar executives have psychological as well as physical training; it's not to give them a break, but to increase their ability to perform at their peak during times of high stress and intense competition. Those who meditate regularly are able to do the mental or cognitive equivalent of patting their head and rubbing their tummy. They can perform self-evaluation or self-referral tasks while also performing external tasks such as running down the basketball court at high speed while slowing down the picture mentally in order to breathe, focus, and make the three pointers while all the time having increased situational awareness of the other players. They become the cat, vibrantly aware, alert, relaxed, not only with their brain, but also due to increased connectivity and bodily awareness, of every cell in their body.

The perception of pain also changes in meditators. While situational awareness and awareness of body, sensations of hot, cold, sharp, dull, pressure and pain are much more developed in the meditators, they do not suffer. Think of it as "that is sharp so I will quickly move away from it," and "That is hot as I approach it so I will not stay here long enough to get burned." Like catching the ball before you even know cognitively it is coming or shifting out of the way of the door as it swings open even before you realized it was opening behind you, there is an uncanny situational awareness which involves the whole of your being, coherently working together and sharing information at speeds higher than can be consciously processed. This is why Samurai warriors and martial art masters practice meditation and mindfulness, to not only increase awareness and peak performance, but to continually rebuild the body after battle, sparring, or competition.

Meditation, breathing, and mindfulness have been practiced for thousands of years in countries such as China, Japan, and India where longevity and health into old age is well known. Sadly, as younger generations in these countries adopt the Western lifestyle, they too are seeing a higher incidence of chronic disease and chronic pain similar to their Western counterparts.

While attending the "Journey into Healing" conference, co-sponsored by the University of California, San Diego, Scripps Center for Integrative Medicine, and the Chopra Center in Encinitas California, I heard Dr. Dean Ornish speak. Dr. Ornish is a cardiologist, founder, and president of the non-profit Preventive Medicine Research Institute and Clinical Professor of Medicine at UCSF and at UCSD. He and his colleagues at the Preventive Medicine Research Institute performed research over thirty-five years, which is now published in the highest level of peer-reviewed journals. They showed that in multiple research groups, from different parts of the country, in just TWELVE WEEKS, with a combination of an anti-inflammatory diet, moderate exercise and mindfulness, patients were able to change the function of over five hundred genes, turning off disease-producing genes and turning on disease-preventing genes! They were able to turn off genes involved in prostate and breast cancer, heart disease, inflammation, and many other genes associated with chronic pain and chronic disease. In addition, telomerase (the enzymes which prepare telomeres which protect the ends of the chromosomes of our DNA and determine how long we live) was increased by 30% in just twelve weeks. At one and five years, the coronary arteries of the study individuals had opened up significantly and they had a 300% increase in blood flow to the heart on average, without surgery, angioplasty or medications! The coronary heart disease of the control group, who did not change their lifestyle but had the best of modern medications, surgery, and angioplasty, in contrast, continued to worsen at one and five years. (7)

Because of the high-level of evidence produced from these studies, the Dr. Ornish Program was approved by a bi-partisan house of Congress to be covered by Medicare, and now is covered by many health insurance companies in the United States for patients with chronic heart disease. But just as it works for severe chronic heart disease, could the same program work for chronic pain?

Reversing Chronic Pain

One of the most important books, *Healing Back Pain Naturally,* that I recommend to my chronic pain patients is written by an Orthopedic Surgeon, Dr. Art

Bernstein. A common question I am asked by patients is: "Am I just going to get worse and eventually need surgery?" or "another surgery?" and I tell them about Dr. Bernstein.

By the time he was thirty-five years old, Dr. Bernstein had undergone three back surgeries, including a fusion. After his surgeries, he continued to suffer from chronic back pain and a reliance on strong pain medications. He had been an athlete but was no longer able to surf or engage in sports. After learning from mind body experts and pioneers such as Harvard's Dr. Herbert Benson about techniques that help to heal and rebuild the body, he was able to give up his reliance on opioids and return to an active lifestyle. He went on to develop a "Back to Life" program in Hawaii where he has his practice. His program and book have helped countless patients recover from incapacitating back pain by giving them the simple tools for healing and developing a lifestyle which works holistically to change unhealthy lifestyle patterns. (8)

A third reference that I give to my patients to help them develop hope that even they can heal, no matter how severe their pain, no matter how many parts of their body hurt constantly, no matter how much they are suffering, is the website and workbook by Dr. Michael Moskowitz and Dr. Marla Golden, which allows them to understand how profoundly we can transform our own health and heal from chronic pain by utilizing tools as simple as mental imagery and our own five senses.

After suffering from progressive neck pain which became incapacitating over the course of fifteen years,

Dr. Moskowitz studied thousands of pages of scientific evidence which demonstrated that chronic pain is processed in more than twelve areas of the brain and these areas also have other functions. In one of these areas, for example, we process mental imaging. While chronic pain takes over or dominates these areas over time, especially when we ruminate or think constantly about our pain, by creating peaceful, enjoyable mental imagery, we can take back the area which chronic pain has stolen and "shrink the map" of chronic pain in the brain.

Dr. Moskowitz was able to reverse his own severe chronic pain using these techniques. Then he and Dr. Golden developed techniques that help their patients, many who have been on disability due to chronic pain for up to thirty years, to "shrink the map of pain" in the brain. By using the power of positive sights, sounds, smells, touch, and thoughts, also processed in the areas of the brain which are taken over by chronic pain, we can take back the geography which was stolen and help the body and mind to heal from chronic pain. Patients can purchase their workbook or access it on their website. Dr. Moskowitz and Dr. Golden have made their workbook freely available online. They also speak at conferences to educate patients and health care professionals alike as to how we can become our own neuroscientists. Dr. Moskowitz teaches the patient to use the brain to heal the body and Dr. Golden teaches them to use the body to heal the brain. (9)

To help patients overcome the erroneous idea that the adult brain is "set" and cannot be healed, they give all of their patients Norman Doidge, MD's book, *The*

Brain's Way of Healing, to help them understand the amazing capacity of the human brain and body to heal at any age. One of the chapters from Dr. Doidge's first book, *The Brain That Changes Itself*, tells the story of Dr. Taub, who after years of research into the workings of the nervous system, developed a remarkable system, which allows patients who have suffered from illness such as stroke, traumatic brain injury, brain tumors, or multiple sclerosis to re-wire their brain by learning to use the affected parts of their body rather than relying on the less affected parts. Language or limb function can be restored utilizing these methods REGARDLESS of the number of years that have lapsed from the time of the injury or illness. Brain imaging studies show changes in the brain that mirror the improvement in function of the body or speech. (10, 11)

When my patients ask me why they have not heard of these things, I tell them, "Because as physicians, we do not learn this in medical school, or even in college (unless we study graduate level physics and nonlinear mathematics)." Our current system of Western conventional medicine is based on the science of the 1400s to the 1700s. At that time, the great scientists of the scientific revolution including Descartes, Bacon, Galileo, Kepler, and Sir Isaac Newton, believed in the separation of mind and body. They believed that the human body and the universe could, like a clock, be understood by breaking them down into their smallest components using a scientific, analytical approach. This approach was founded on the idea that the mind, emotions, and the body could be studied and treated completely separately. The structure of our current medical system reflects this approach. One specialist treats your feet, another your brain, another your mind and emotions, another your eyes, still another your heart, yet another your liver, etc. Each fix or replaces that part as if it were a piece of a broken clock, without regard for the whole human being.

Although the ideas and concepts of the scientific revolution have served us well and have helped us to develop many advances in science and medicine, with more advanced techniques tools and mathematical concepts and proofs, Nobel prize winning scientists of the 1800s to the present have advanced our understanding of living systems and the universe.

Although most of us have heard terms such as "Quantum Mechanics," "Chaos Theory," and Heisenberg's "Uncertainty principle," most of us are unaware that these concepts also apply to living beings and ecological systems, and not just to subatomic particle physics and cosmology. Certainly, these concepts are not taught in medical school. The implications of these concepts, proven time and again through rigorous advanced scientific methodology, are that we cannot separate mind, body, emotions, or the spiritual aspect of human beings. The new physics shows us that the universe, from the microscopic to the macrocosm, the smallest to the largest part, is a whole, and that the whole is greater than the sum of its parts. This is because the parts are in relationship to each other.

Quantum physics, quantum biology, and nonlinear mathematics give us a qualitative, not a quantitative sense of reality. They reveal to us that if we analyze or break the whole into parts, we destroy what makes it a living being, an ecosystem, a living universe. Since the observer is a part of the whole, our very perceptions, questions, and how we ask them affect the whole, the answer that we obtain, the view that we see. So how can we change our questions and the way we see the world? (12)

Exercise for Expanding to an Unlimited Mindset

Sit in a quiet place where you will not be disturbed. If necessary, support your back with pillows so that you are sitting comfortably with your back and neck in a neutral position, feet flat on the floor in front of you, hands resting on your thighs. Observe your breathing, relax your breathing, allow your body to relax starting at the top of your head and slowly moving down to your face, neck, shoulders, arms, hands, back, chest, abdomen, hips, thighs, legs, and feet. Keeping your eyes softly closed, imagine or think of a healing place or sanctuary of your own creation where you can be transported by *Star Trek* or other advanced futuristic teleportation or by magical beings or animal guardians. This place can be a single room, your own island, secret estate, planet, space ship, luxury submarine, or cave in the Andes or in Tibet. Imagine that you have everything there that you need to heal. You have wise beings from the past or the present, master healers from any age, country, or planet, music, sounds, healing foods and herbs, gardens, forests, birds, and other healing creatures. Imagine the colors, surroundings, sounds, people (you can have silence, then rooms and spaces where you can meet with a friend or friends and loved ones here or from the past, for as short or long of time as you would like). You can be transported to a private beach, lake, healing natural springs, or any other place that brings you a feeling of peace, joy, and well-being. You can ask for anything that you feel would bring you relief, healing, well-being, happiness, and joy. You can ask your assistants for any information which you need. Relax and observe. If you have intruding thoughts that are fear-based or limitation-based, just notice and thank them, gently let them go, and return to your healing place.

You can return to this place at any time. You can keep it the same or modify it to your desire. When you are satisfied with your journey, slowly return to the present time and place.

Chapter 3

OUR EMOTIONS AND CHRONIC PAIN

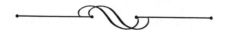

"The word I would stress in regard to this integrated system is 'network,'"... In thinking about these matters, then, it might make more sense to emphasize the perspective of psychology rather than of neuroscience. For the term psycho clearly conveys the study of mind, and perhaps mind is the information flowing among all of these bodily parts, and that may be what mind is. A mind is composed of information, and it has a physical substrate, which is the body and the brain, and it also has another immaterial substrate that has to do with information flowing around. Maybe mind is what holds the network together."
– Candace Pert, PhD (1)

While in private pain management practice in Florida, I was on call every other night and every other weekend to respond to requests by other physicians to assist with uncontrolled pain for patients whom they had admitted to three of the local hospitals where I held privileges. My partners and I were frequently called to see patients who had been admitted to the psychiatric unit. That is expected, because, as I explained in the last chapter, chronic pain and mental health disorders such as chronic anxiety and depression are co-processed in the same networks of the nervous system. Thus, the chronic pain population has a much larger percentage of patients with chronic mental health disorders, and the mental health population has a much larger percentage of chronic pain than the general population as a whole.

One evening, as I entered the locked psychiatric unit and was looking for the patient whom I had been consulted to evaluate by one of the psychiatrists, I found her in the visitor's area. She was a tiny girl in her early twenties. Her young, handsome husband was cradling her in his arms and their precious little boy, who looked to be about four years old, stood next to her holding her hand. I called her name and they gave her kisses as she left with me for the exam room. She had been admitted for a series of electroconvulsive therapy (ECT) sessions for treatment resistant depression. I had been called to assist with her severe migraine, which was persistent due to the need for patients undergoing ECT to come off of all medications that prevent seizures. These included her migraine preventive medication and her anti-anxiety medications.

After performing nerve blocks and trigger point injections to alleviate her migraine and listening to her lament the loss of her anti-anxiety medication, I thought for a moment, at a loss for what to say. Then I remembered the touching scene that I had seen of her being lovingly held by her husband and son. I told her of how I had observed them and then said, "I think that we as human beings underestimate the power we have to create our own sense of well-being. I was wondering, if any drug which you have taken has ever made you feel as good as when someone you love comes into the room?" A gentle smile swept across her face and tears welled up in her eyes in response to my posit.

I was not alone in pondering the effects of our emotions and our thoughts on pain and our overall health. As I researched the scientific literature on thoughts, emotions, and pain, I learned just how critical our thoughts and emotions are to not only feeling pain in any one moment, but for the development of chronic pain.

In the next few years, multiple studies would be published in both European and American medical journals, which analyzed dozens of high-level studies performed over the previous thirty years. All of the studies showed that certain psychological or emotional factors were more predictive of not only developing back pain, but of developing chronic low back pain (the number one pain complaint in the US and other industrialized countries). Not only did these factors predict who would most likely develop low back pain, but they predicted it with much more significance than did factors related to occupation, medical diagnosis, general health, fitness or strength. (2, 3)

These important thoughts and emotions which predicted that someone would be more likely to develop both acute and chronic low back pain were: fear avoidance (being afraid to do things such as exercise or social activities for fear of making your pain worse or injuring yourself), depressive thoughts and catastrophizing (thinking of the very worst thing that could happen then continually worrying about it), and passive coping styles (depending on something or someone outside of yourself, which is the opposite of self-reliance).

Fear avoidance was found to be associated with physical deconditioning, taking on the identity of being sick, negative emotions such as chronic sadness, worry, fear and anger, and withdrawing from friends and family. All of these were most predictive of long-term disability.

But, how can we change the way we think, and what is so important about being self-reliant? These same scientists actually showed that with teaching patients self-reliance and how to change destructive thought and behavior patterns, they were able to prevent the development of persistent low back pain! In regard to the importance of self-reliance, according to just one of many studies on the health benefits associated with self-reliance and self-regulation, after observing 5,716 middle-aged adults with equal risk factors for chronic disease over fifteen years, researchers found that those who had self-reliance, at the end of the fifteen-year observation period, had a fifty percent LOWER incidence of chronic disease and death than those with poor self-reliance. (4)

Think of learning self-reliance as learning how to ride a bicycle. At first it is hard to keep the bicycle going where you want it to go. The wheel turns to the right, so in order to not fall down, the child learns to turn the wheel to the left, then to the right. Initially, the oscillations are quite large ... but in time, as the child gains greater skill ... the oscillations diminish and are barely perceptible.

It sometimes takes a while to learn how to self-regulate ... like riding a bike. In human beings, homeostasis is defined as the tendency toward a relatively stable equilibrium between interdependent elements, especially as maintained by physiological processes. Sounds like learning to ride a bike, right?

Physiologically then, self-regulation is associated with a balance between the sympathetic and parasympathetic components of the autonomic nervous system (which we talked about in chapter 2). This balance is apparent in individuals with high heart rate variability, which is a predictor of physiologic resilience and self-regulation.

Humans, as all living organisms, must constantly adapt to stressors in order to maintain a state of homeostasis. Allostasis is the ongoing adaptive efforts of the body to maintain homeostasis in response to environmental stressors.

Lack of resilience, or a persistent, large scale insult may result in dysregulation or imbalance in the immune, endocrine, nervous, and musculoskeletal systems. Those with the most practice in self-regulation are most likely to be able to get back to equilibrium or balance after such a trauma, illness, or injury.

According to Keith Griffin of "Healthtrax," an insurance plan that rewards employees for healthy living, just like learning to ride a bicycle it may take a while for people to learn to make healthy decisions and to help them establish a preventive rather than a reactive approach to healthcare. At first, health care expenses may go up as previously undiagnosed conditions are stabilized. Subsequently however, costs have been shown to decline progressively as patients become more autonomous and self-regulating.

Complementary and Alternative Medicine and Self-Regulation

During my two years of private practice in pain management in 1999-2000, there was great concern about the under-treatment of pain in America and both physicians and national health care organizations made a large effort to liberalize the treatment of those suffering from chronic pain with opioids. Throughout the next decade however, it became apparent that as the number of prescriptions of opioids increased, so did the deaths associated with opioid overdose. This continued until deaths from opioids overtook deaths from automobile accidents as the number one cause of death in young people in the eighteen- to thirty-five-year-old age range.

At the same time, Military and Veteran Association Hospital Physicians were also finding an increase in accidental deaths from polypharmacy and opioids. The most important finding was that despite an increase in the prescription of opioids and polypharmacy, this approach did not improve the function or overall well-being of patients with chronic pain. In fact, recent studies showed that higher opioid doses for chronic pain are associated with multiple poor outcomes compared to patients not taking opioids or patients on lower doses. These include falls, fractures, opioid overdose, greater pain intensity, worse functioning, worse quality of life, poorer self-efficacy for managing pain, greater fear avoidance, and more health care utilization. (5)

Although in the setting of acute injury and pain, opioids serve a useful purpose to reduce pain and suffering during the initial healing phase, many physicians and patients do not understand that, simply put, the human body is much more intelligent than the pill. We take the opioids, which act on the opioid receptors, which are on the descending part of the pain pathway. Meanwhile, the areas of our brain that register pain coming up the ascending pain pathway say, "You are not fooling me with that fake opioid stuff. I still have pain signals coming up here so I'm going to turn down my opioid receptors." The patient then takes more opioids and the body again turns down the receptors. If the physician and patient do not understand this and escalate or increase the opioid dose in attempt to relieve the pain, since another side effect of the opioid is to decrease the rate and depth of breathing, at one point during the escalation, which is difficult to predict, the patient falls asleep and simply does not wake up.

This innate characteristic of opioids is called tolerance. This means that over time, the same dose of opioids will no longer be effective. Even in those patients who do not suffer from overdose, the negative effects of opioids have been shown to adversely affect overall health and well-being in chronic pain by suppressing immune function, reducing testosterone in men and estrogen in women, and causing depression and weight gain. Also, the cells in our nervous system which make our own internally manufactured "endorphins," which provide us with a pain relief and a sense of wellbeing in times of stress, die off when we take opioids over a long time (the use it or lose it principle – our body says, "there's a lot of that stuff floating around so I don't have to make it anymore") and thus patients on chronic opioids will often develop wide-spread pain and sensitivity, the exact opposite of what they are trying to achieve.

Because of the growing awareness of both the limitations and risks associated with the long-term use of opioids in chronic pain, and the growing research which reveals the importance of self-regulation, resiliency and autonomic nervous system regulation, both military and civilian pain specialists and organizations have increased their use of evidence-based complementary and alternative approaches as these help with both autonomic nervous system regulation and the building of self-efficacy. However, the problem remains that many of these approaches are not covered by insurance plans and thus are not available to large numbers of patients.

In response to the opioid crisis, Congress mandated that an integrated, interdisciplinary, and educational approach be developed in addition to guidelines regarding the safe use of opioids. In 2009, I was invited to be a member of Integrative Medicine panel of The Army Surgeon General's 2010 Pain Task Force and helped with the adoption of guidelines for the utilization of the top six evidence-based complementary modalities for chronic pain within the Army's Integrative Pain Management Clinics.

In these clinics, in addition to conventional Interventional Pain Management and pharmacologic approaches, complementary modalities are available including: acupuncture, cognitive behavior therapy, chiropractic therapy, medical massage, and Yoga Nidra. The US Navy and the US Air Force Surgeon Generals also oversaw development of integrative, interdisciplinary approaches to pain management in these services with dramatic increases in the availability of wellness approaches and programs.

One of the tenets of the Pain Task Force was the emphasis on helping service members and their families develop self-reliance and resiliency (due to the association of resiliency and well-being). The ideal model for development of self-efficacy illustrated the transition from passive reliance on others for care to self-care. For example, a patient should be encouraged to move from receiving acupuncture to also performing self-help acupressure, from attending a Qigong class to also performing self-guided Qigong with the use of a video at home, from obtaining chiropractic manipulation to also performing self-corrective exercise.

The civilian pain community was also undergoing a similar reassessment of their approach to pain management. According to the International Association for the Study of Pain's clinical update on Integrative Medicine, a Holistic Model of Care: "Prevailing pain-management practices, which include liberal use of surgery, interventions, and drugs, are not adequately addressing the growing cohort of chronic pain patients. The reports on pain prepared by the Institute of Medicine in 2011 and the U.S. Army Surgeon General's Pain Management Task Force both concluded that tinkering with the prevailing system of care will not address the problem."

These reports speak of the culture change needed to address an inadequate system. "Military medicine has been very specific in its prescriptive recommendations: flip the therapeutic order, and rather than beginning with drugs or costly and risky interventions and surgeries, begin with yoga, massage, chiropractic care, or acupuncture."

The report goes on to elaborate: "Recognition of the innate capacity of people to heal through self-care strategies is a cornerstone of IM (Integrative Medicine) and this approach empowers patients to assume control over their health. The practitioner is present as a guide to partner with the patient in a healing journey. The existing time-based fee-for-service model, the over-reliance on technology, and the inability of the establishment medical system to treat chronic disease adequately are also reasons patients turn to CAM and IM practitioners. Perhaps the most compelling reason to embrace integrative pain strategies is to mitigate the risk to patients. Awareness is growing of serious adverse effects of medications, including the escalating rates of inadvertent overdoses from prescription opioids and the development of opioid tolerance and opioid- induced hyperalgesia. The statistics on non-steroidal anti-inflammatory drugs (NSAIDs) show that deaths in the

United States from these drugs now exceed deaths from HIV/AIDS." (6)

It is important to emphasize that the report does not advocate lack of reliance on allopathic medicine or on pharmacologic approaches when needed and appropriate. The report does note however, that many of us have become less than self-reliant. According to the Institute of Medicine 2011 report "Relieving Pain in America: Blueprint for Transforming Prevention, Care, Education and Research," "our current system lacks resources for education of both patients and health care providers as to the nature and causes of pain, methods to prevent and treat acute and chronic pain, the importance of self-reliance and self-help methods for the management of acute exacerbations of chronic pain." (7)

As a medical acupuncturist, during my frequent review of the scientific literature on the underlying mechanisms of acupuncture, I found that it was becoming evident that, according to numerous studies, acupuncture was effective in treating so many different health disorders, because it works to harmonize the underlying systems of the body such as the autonomic nervous system, neuroendocrine system, and the immune system. Using the same underlying mechanisms, complementary and alternative self-help modalities such as mediation, Taiichi, Jin Shin Jyutsu, self-help, yoga, and Qigong can restore balance to these underlying systems of the body. They also increase self-reliance and resiliency, as they can be used at home, during travel, and in-between visits to health care practitioners as a preventative measure, to maintain health, and to treat pain exacerbations.

Heart Rate Variability and Wellbeing/Rapid self-regulation

While I was stationed in Newport, Rhode Island and was looking for answers to help my patients with intractable pain and associated anxiety, panic disorders, insomnia, and depression I learned about the research performed by the nonprofit HeartMath Institute system which is used by many Fortune 500 companies, the military, hospitals, and schools to help their executives, service members, patients, and students regain their health and a sense of well-being and become self-regulating and resilient. Based on abundant research showing that high heart rate variation is associated with increased health and longevity they teach individuals and groups how to develop high heart rate variability through simple exercises such as the "Freeze Frame," "Cut through, "and "Heart Lock in" methods. These methods retrain the way we process and react to stressful situations, thoughts and emotions.

It is well known that how we perceive and respond to information emotionally affects many centers in the brain, which regulate the immune system, autonomic nervous system, and hormonal systems. These systems are in constant communication with neural networks in the heart. If we see the world as hostile, threatening, and stressful, we produce increases in stress hormones such as cortisol, which over time, cause chronic pain, heart disease, elevated blood sugar, bone loss, poor immune system function, fat accumulation, and a decrease in brain function. Whereas emotions that dampen the stress response, such as appreciation and gratitude, are associated with an increase in the hormone precursor DHEA. High levels of DHEA are associated with health, recovery, and longevity.

One of the first studies published by the HeartMath Institute was "The Impact of a New Emotional Self-Management Program on Stress, Emotions, Heart Rate Variability DHEA and Cortisol." After a one-day training session and thirty minutes a day of practice at least five days per week for one month, the research subjects (but not the control group) were found to have a 23% *decrease* in salivary cortisol and a 100% *increase* in DHEA. The experimental group (but not the control group), after just four weeks, was found to have a significant increase in caring and vigor and a significant decrease in guilt, hostility, stress, anxiety, and "over-caring" (constant anxiety and worrying).

In another early HeartMath Institute study, *just five minutes of care or compassion* were associated with an increase in immune system markers (which lasted several hours). In contrast, *after five minutes of anger*, there was a temporary elevation of immune system markers followed by a significant drop in immune markers that lasted for several hours. The drop in immune system markers was also associated with heart rate increases and negative mood, along with numerous physical symptoms including headache, dry mouth, and muscle pains (which also lasted for several hours after the experience of anger).

Another important HeartMath study, which I often relate to my active duty service Marines and other combat service members is a study involving the Santa Clara California Police Department. Before the HeartMath "Freeze Frame "training (a four step process involving: recognition of the state of negative emotion, breathing while focusing on the area of the heart, visualizing a scene or person which evokes feelings of gratitude and calm, then finding a positive rather than negative response to the current feeling or situation), when the police officers encountered a situation such as ... opens door ... sees man with gun ... guns go up ... shots fired ... take down ... cuffing ... , it took, on average, *105 minutes* for the police officer's heart rate to return to normal. After one month of practicing HeartMath's four step Freeze Frame training, it took an average of *120-150 seconds* for their heart rate and blood pressure to return to normal! In addition, according to the results of a psychological and performance assessment and semi-structured interview conducted after the training, the officers stated that additional benefits from the training included:

- Increased awareness and self-management of stress reactions
- Greater confidence, balance, and clarity under acute stress
- Quicker physiological and psychological recalibration following acute stress
- Improved work performance
- Reduced competition, improved communication, and greater cooperation within work teams

- Reduced distress, anger, sadness, and fatigue
- Reduced sleeplessness and physical stress symptoms
- Increased peacefulness and vitality
- Improved listening and relationships with family (8, 9).

Emotions and the Brain

So how could the way the brain processes emotions cause or reduce physical stress symptoms, fatigue, aches and pains, and other physical symptoms in the body? I found out the answer to this question when I learned about the research of Candace Pert, PhD and Michael Ruff, PhD from my niece, who has a master's in acupuncture and Chinese medicine.

Dr. Candace Pert is best known for her discovery of the opioid receptor during her doctorate research at John Hopkins University in 1979. She later became section head of Brain Biochemistry at the National Institute of Health and still later, Professor of Medicine at Georgetown Medical School.

What she found during her studies of the biochemistry of the brain was that the same chemicals that transmit information to the emotional and thought centers of the *brain are also distributed throughout the body* (a fact that neither I nor any of the medical colleagues whom I have queried were taught in medical school). Dr. Pert explains:

> *"My argument is that the three classic disciplines*
> *of neuroscience, endocrinology, and immunology,*
> *with their various organs-the brain (which is the*

*key organ that the neuroscientists study), the glands,
and the immune system (consisting of the spleen,
the bone marrow, the lymph nodes, and of course
the distributed cells throughout the body)-that these
three areas are actually joined to each other in a
bidirectional network of communication and that the
information "carriers" are the neuropeptides. There
are well-studied physiological substrates showing that
communication exists in both directions for every
single one of these areas and their organs."*

– Candace Pert, PhD

Dr. Pert argued that the feelings we have in the pit of our stomach, our muscles, and throughout our bodies, are the results of the chemicals which are generated by our thoughts and emotions, that these chemicals not only have receptors in our nervous system, but throughout our entire body! In her own words:

*"The last point I am going to make about the
neuropeptides is an astounding one I think. As we
have seen, neuropeptides are signaling molecules.
They send messages all over the body (including the
brain). Of course, to have such a communications
network, you need components that can talk to each
other and listen to each other. In the situation we
are discussing here, the components that "talk" are
the neuropeptides, and the components that "hear"
are the neuropeptide receptors. How can this be? …
Why does order rather than chaos reign? It has to do
with the specificity, the selectivity of the receptors,
not their direct wiring, not neuron to neuron."*

*"I note in passing that the receptors are quite
capable of changing their conformations within
the cell membranes ... so rapid that it's hard to
tell whether it is in one state or another at a given
moment in time ... , receptors have both a wave-
like and a particle character, and it is important to
note that information can be stored in the form of
time spent in different states."*
– Candace Pert PhD

So, here, Dr. Pert is referring to a "Quantum State." We are both energy and matter all at once, mind, body, and spirit at once at the level where conscious and unconscious states intersect; subconscious perceptions and conscious thought affect the state of feeling and the long-term state of health or chronic disease of the brain and body alike, and at once.

But there is even more that we must learn in order to understand how our conscious and unconscious beliefs affect our perceptions and create health and well-being or pain and disease. Enter stage left ... the Placebo and the Nocebo effects.

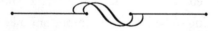

Gate Theory Exercise:

To turn down the firing of the pain fibers, simply rub or place pressure on the painful area. This activates non-painful sensory fibers that will "close the gate" and inhibit pain signal firing up the ascending pain pathway. A TENS unit (transcutaneous electrical nerve stimulation unit) works by the same gate theory mechanism.

HeartMath Freeze Frame Exercise:

1. Recognize or become aware that you are in an emotional state of anger, fear, panic, anxiety, stress. Freeze the frame.

2. Start taking slow, deep breaths and focus on the area around the heart to recall emotional feelings of appreciation and gratitude. While shifting your thoughts away from the disturbed, fearful, angry thoughts, keep focusing on your breathing and your heart for at least ten seconds or more.

3. Recall a positive, peaceful, fun event or place from your life or imagination and re-experience this place or feeling of peace, calm, or fun.

4. Now, think of a positive solution to the current situation that would minimize current and future anxiety and stress.

5. Pay attention to what your heart tells you in regard to the above solution as a way to decrease your reactive emotions and thoughts and use a more common sense, effective solution.

6. An example of the above would be the situation where you are stuck in a traffic jam and are going to be late for an important meeting or to pick up your child. You catch yourself swearing at the driver who cut you off and pounding on your car horn. You then freeze the frame, take a time out, shift your focus away from your thoughts and racing mind, disturbed emotional state, focus on your breath and on the area of your heart to help change the focus

to feelings of appreciation and gratitude (which remember, cause a decrease in cortisol and inflammation and an increase in DHEA and immune system function as well as improved sense of well-being). Think of an image or memory of something fun or peaceful or meaningful in a positive way to you. Attempt to re-experience this positive time or event. Now think of a positive solution (for example: get on the Bluetooth and call work or the school and let them know that you are in a traffic jam and will be there as soon as possible, then turn on music which makes you feel relaxed/good). (10)

PART TWO

Chapter 4

THE POWER OF BELIEF

"When you change the way you look at things, the things you look at change."
– Physicist Max Planck

I n 2011, I attended an integrative medicine conference in San Diego, hosted by Scripps Center for Integrative Medicine. The famous country-western singer Naomi Judd held a special speaking event and book signing for her best-selling book, *Naomi's Breakthrough Guide,* on one of the evenings of the conference. She was there to raise funds for the Naval Hospital Camp Pendleton's Healing Touch program for the US Marines suffering from PTSD. The program had been started as a joint research project between Scripps Center for Integrative Medicine and staff at The Holistic Health Center at Naval Hospital Camp Pendleton. After the study was completed, there continued to be high demand for the gentle restorative complementary medicine approach, so Naomi Judd was here to raise money to continue Healing Touch for the US Marines with PTSD at Naval Hospital Camp Pendleton.

Naomi got up, looked around at the large audience, and said, "I bet you can't guess what you and I have in common!" Several hands shot up. "We both have red hair," one man replied. "We are both from Kentucky." She shook her head in response to each of these, and when everyone had given up, she replied, "We all know more about me than we know about you!" She then went on to say to the audience that we are a celebrity culture and love to read about stars and athletes and other celebrities but take little time to understand who we are as individuals … to learn about ourselves.

She told about her journey from being lonely, broke, sick, aimless, and desperate, to having a happy marriage and family life, being financially secure and healing from chronic disease. Her story and her book are about "using some Windex on the window to your soul," to look at the beliefs we have which have gotten us to where we are, and how by changing our beliefs, we can change our lives. She says, in the section of her book called, "When You Change Your Mind You Change Your World," that, "Every expert I spoke to, whether a doctor, behavioral scientist, molecular biologist, physicist or biochemist, agreed on one thing: nothing can get better in our lives until we decide to change the way that we're thinking about a problem."

Later in her book, Naomi quotes psychiatrist and best-selling author Dr. M. Scott Peck, author of *The Road Less Traveled,* who said that, "Sooner or later, if people are to be healed, they must learn that the entirety of one's adult life is a series of personal choices. If they can accept this totally, then they become free. The extent that they cannot accept this, they will forever feel themselves victims."

The wonderful thing about awareness is that it leads us to examine how the things we believe, often at a level we may not have ever realized, either imprison, trap us, or liberate us.

Placebo, Nocebo and Meaning

> *"Some patients, though conscious that their condition is perilous, recover their health simply through their contentment with the goodness of their physician."*
> – Hippocrates

Our beliefs and the meaning that we ascribe to the events and people in our lives have been found to profoundly affect our response to medication, surgery, and our ability to heal. The scientific name for this phenomenon is the placebo effect (if the response is in the positive direction) and the nocebo effect (if it is in the negative direction).

Placebo in Latin means, "I shall be pleasing or acceptable" and is attributed to belief and expectancy on the part of the patient, on the part of the caregiver, and generated by a relationship between the patient and the caregiver. For example, if the relationship between a physician and a patient is based on trust, acceptance, and confidence, studies show that the patient is more likely to have a positive response to medication prescribed or procedures performed by that physician. On the contrary, if the patient does not have faith or trust in a physician, he or she is less likely to have a positive effect from treatments offered by that physician and more likely to even have a negative effect.

An example of a placebo effect is a patient's positive response to a medication that has been advertised as being a major breakthrough drug for treating their condition. Studies have reported a drop in response to "old medications" when "new" medications for the same treatment are advertised. In fact, suggestion and belief is so powerful that in one study, when patients were given ipecac, a medication known to produce vomiting, but were told that it was to treat their nausea, the majority of the patients experienced relief of their nausea symptoms. In another study, the "nocebo" effect was observed when patients who were allergic to lacquer were exposed to chestnut and told that it was lacquer. Fifty-one percent of the patients had allergic responses, believing that they had been exposed to a something to which they were allergic. (1)

Henry Beecher, MD, from Massachusetts Hospital reported in 1955 that the placebo response occurred on average during experiments in up to 30% of patients. However, Herbert Benson MD, the renowned Harvard Cardiologist and Mind Body researcher, along with his colleague David McCallie Jr. MD, reviewed the response of patients to past unproven medical therapies such as cobra venom, and showed that when the therapies were used and believed in, they were 70-90%

effective. "However, when the physicians began to doubt that the treatments worked, their effectiveness dropped to 30-40%" (2).

In a recent article entitled *Reconstructing the Placebo Effect and Finding the Meaning Effect,* the authors remind us that it is not the sham pill or sham surgery which causes the placebo effect, rather it is the ability of the human being to respond in either a positive or negative way to those things, events, procedures or words which have meaning to them. They give the account of a study where college students were asked to participate in a study of two new drugs. They were given packets of either one or two red pills or one or two blue pills (which were inert with no medicinal properties). A questionnaire given to the students after they took the pills revealed that the students believed that the red pills were stimulants and the blue pills were tranquilizers and that taking two pills produced a more powerful effect than taking one pill. These responses mirrored previously tested beliefs in the meaning of colors and numbers (red means" hot," "up," "active," "danger," and blue means "cool," "quiet," "down" and two means "more than one"). (3)

The placebo effect has been studied extensively in researching how patients respond to and heal from surgery, and why some patients need more medication or develop chronic pain and others don't. In a study of the placebo effect on pain, patients were given either a cursory and cold, or warm and detailed preoperative visit by their anesthesiologist. Those who had the warm and detailed preoperative visit were found to use 50% less pain medication and were discharged from the hospital an average of 2.7 days earlier than those patients who had a cursory and cold preoperative visit. (4)

J.D. Salinger is a famous author who is admired for his great novels. The best known is *Catcher in the Rye*, a coming of age story that was required reading in middle schools for decades throughout much of the US. In WWII he was a soldier in some of the bloodiest battles of WWII. His daughter, Margaret Salinger, in her book *Dream Catcher*, tells how the events he witnessed and suffered during the war affected him for the rest of his life and became a part of his mannerisms, his relationships, and the characters in his books. Though the events of WWII never left him, he became one of the most successful American novelists of the 20th century and wove with his mind and spirit, changed as they were by events of the war, stories and characters that continue to impact generations.

Just as removing a strand of an intricate spider's web would affect the structure of the entire web, the body, mind, and spirit are each affected by wounds of the body or mind or spirit. Indeed, functional Magnetic Resonance Imaging (fMRI) shows that the brain of a patient with a chronic pain compared with that of a patient without chronic pain will have dramatically different patterns of activation throughout the complex centers which are activated in chronic pain, when both are exposed to a painful stimulus.

More recently, as technology has advanced, clinical and neuroscientists such as Sean Mackie, MD and his team of researchers at Stanford Medical Center are researching the astounding ability of patients with chronic pain to alternatively increase or decrease the activation of the main centers in the brain where pain is processed. Using real time functional Magnetic Resonance Imaging (rtfMRI) Neurofeedback, patients are given examples of thoughts, emotions or visualization strategies which were successful when used by other subjects in increasing or decreasing activation in these brain centers.

The patients were found to be most successful if they were given leeway to then devise their own unique approach or strategy. As they increased the activation of these brain centers, their pain increased, and as they decreased the activation, they were able to drop their pain by more than 44%. These changes were shown to persist for the duration of the study period. The researchers were also able to reproduce these changes in pain with patients who were using the same techniques and who were not able to visualize their brain using the rtfMRI. Interestingly, in one rtfMRI study, the researchers told patients who suffered from chronic pain that they had stopped giving them the powerful intravenous opioid that they had been receiving for their pain. As they did so, the pain centers were strongly activated in the brain and the patient's pain became severe, even though, in reality, they were still receiving the same dose of intravenous opioid. It had not been turned off at all, yet the belief that it had been resulted not only in an increase in pain, but in a visible activation of the pain centers in the brain. (5)

How can our thoughts and emotions be that powerful?

"Perhaps all the dragons in our lives are princesses who are only waiting to see us act, just once, with beauty and courage. Perhaps everything that frightens us is in its deepest essence, something helpless that wants our love."

– Reiner Maria Rilke

Exercise:

In the chart below, I will give examples of different meaning responses that are common in patients with chronic pain, some anger and fear-based and passive, and others hopeful and proactive. The list on either side might be, "What does my pain mean to me?" based on your point of view. As an exercise, make your own left-side and right-side lists to examine possible meanings that you have given to your pain, and what messages or meanings it may have for you.

My pain is a punishment for things I have done wrong.	My pain reminds me that I have chosen to believe that I have to push myself beyond my limits in order to be worthy of the love and respect of others. I need to learn to accept myself and care for myself as I would for a little brother or sister, or a dear friend.

My pain is a punishment for others in my life that have hurt me; a testament of the pain they have caused me. If I get better, they will not know how much pain they caused me, how they destroyed my life. Even if it kills me, I will show them how terrible they are, how terribly they hurt me!	By not forgiving others, I am only hurting myself. By healing and creating a life filled with the things, work, and people who inspire me and bring me joy, I show others and myself that we can all have the courage to forgive and to create something beautiful and unique.
As much as I hate my pain, it is a way to not do what others expect of me and which I don't want to do. These are unreasonable things that I should not have to do; things which should not be expected of me or anyone. I always end up doing other people's work since they won't do it or won't do it "right."	My pain has helped me realize that I am living a life chosen for me by others. I am trying so hard to do what I was told I should do, what I thought others expected of me instead of being courageous enough to live my own dream, to just be me. I am learning that this is enough! This is more than enough. Having chronic pain has helped me to set boundaries for myself, take responsibility for the choices that I make and let others be responsible for themselves.

Isn't there a doctor smart enough, a surgeon good enough, a healer gifted enough to heal me? They told me that the last surgeon I went to was one of the best surgeons in the country! I waited four months just to see him. He said that he could fix me. The results from the surgery only lasted six months and then the pain came right back even worse than it was before.

I am realizing that I thought I was immortal. I thought that I could continue to burn the candle at both ends, that I could just lift a 200-pound weight or box anytime without any consequences, that I could eat whatever I wanted to eat as long as I ate something good for me once in a while. I guess this pain is showing me that just like I have to take care of my car if I don't want it to break down, I have to take care of my body, my mind, and my spirit too, or I will continue to break down.

Why won't they give me some pills that work! They just like to see people suffer! They don't care! Can't they see that I am just getting worse? I need to get a wheelchair next time so that they will understand how much pain I am in. They don't understand, it hurts me even to stand up and walk!	I know that I can do this. I might need some help from others along the way, as a bridge while I learn how to take better care of myself, but if other people can heal from chronic pain, I can too. I have done hard things before in life and I can do this too. I am tired of not living. I want to live the life that I dreamed of living. I don't want to live the rest of my life on disability, feeling sorry for myself. I have a lot to give! I don't want to miss out on all of the things I love to do!

I think that many of us, including me, go through life on a treadmill and forget to stop and nourish ourselves, forget to spend time with those who mean most to us, and forget that we are here for just a brief precious time in this life. We forget, or have never discovered who we are, that we are precious too. We forget or have never discovered the priceless gifts that we have to offer to this world.

Agnes DeMille won fame for her choreography of the famous Roger's and Hammerstein's musical *Oklahoma*. In a conversation with her mentor and teacher Martha Graham, she complained bitterly that the critics and public had never recognized her previous work into which she had poured her heart and soul while heaping praise upon a work that she felt was just mediocre. She recounted Martha Graham's reply as the most important thing that anyone had said to her. I feel that it is an essential message for each of us.

"There is a vitality, a life force, an energy, a quickening that is translated through you into action, and because there is only one of you in all of time, this expression is unique. And if you block it, it will never exist through any other medium and it will be lost. The world will not have it.

It is not your business to determine how good it is nor how valuable nor how it compares with other expressions. It is your business to keep it yours clearly and directly, to keep the channel open. You do not even have to believe in yourself or your work. You have to keep yourself open and aware to the urges that motivate you. Keep the channel open."

– Martha Graham

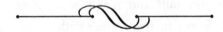

Exercise:

What are the "urges" which motivate you? What are your dreams? What do you love to do? What are your unique talents? What makes you laugh? What makes you tear up at the sheer beauty of it? What has the greatest meaning to you? Write these down! In the next chapter you will find how important they are for creating the life that will help you heal from chronic pain, while also allowing your own dreams to be realized.

Exercise: Getting to Know Who You Are:

As you go through your day, become aware of your thoughts and emotions in regard to simple objects such as your soap, your sheets, the food you eat and other sounds, smells, tastes and textures in your everyday life. When you are engaging in everyday activities, whether at work or at home, take a moment to become aware of your thoughts and feelings. Become of aware of those objects, colors, parts of nature, sounds, tastes, touch, smells, people, movements, and activities that bring you a feeling of satisfaction and joy as well as those that put a knot in your stomach. If it feels right, you may want to ask yourself why you enjoy this or why something is not pleasant or enjoyable to you. Think of this activity as taking a walk in a virgin forest, seeing everything as if for the first time, feeling and smelling and hearing everything with a beginner's mind. Listen to the birds, smell the earth, see the clouds and the shape of the leaves, the shadows and reflections, the wildflowers, as if you had never seen them before. As you come up to a small natural bubbling spring, you feel as if it represents your life, constantly springing up from an unknown source, ever fresh and new. The rocks around the spring can be gently lifted, or not, whenever you are curious, to unlock thoughts, beliefs, and memories which have helped you to get to where you are in your life. As you lift the beautiful rocks, you observe each thought and experience as if you were a stranger to it. Thank it for bringing you to this point in your life. Ask what lessons it might have for you. Then, you can choose to let it go, or gently set the stone down again to revisit this thought or memory at any time in the future which you wish to do so. You can repeat this exercise any time of your choosing. I recommend visiting the virgin forest and spring when you are in a quiet safe undisturbed place, perhaps when you are going to sleep.

Chapter 5

CREATING A CONTEXT FOR HEALING

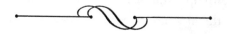

"One thing: you have to walk, and create the way by
your walking; you will not find a ready-made path.
It is not so cheap, to reach to the ultimate realization
of truth. You will have to create the path by walking
yourself; the path is not ready-made, lying there and
waiting for you. It is just like the sky: the birds fly,
but they don't leave any footprints. You cannot follow
them; there are no footprints left behind."

– Osho

I returned home to my parent's ranch with my three-year-old daughter after my divorce. In the deeply religious home and culture which I grew up in, divorce was seen as a deep failure, yet after six years in a violent marriage, I knew that while I could sacrifice my own safety, I could not endanger my child. I had gone to college for two years prior to my marriage and as an eighteen-year-old dreamer, had chosen the fields of speech and drama with an art minor. Now, at age twenty-six, I knew that I needed something more practical and financially reliable than acting in theatre and the occasional modeling for designers to support my daughter and myself.

My research into the job market showed that healthcare was a field with a large demand and reliable income. I had always done well in school, but with a linguist mother and political scientist professor father, I had grown up immersed in literature, history, languages, music, the arts, and theatre. I knew that in the years ahead, I would need to study a curriculum heavy in science. I had "wriggled" out hard science in high school by taking "advanced biology," which did require me to compare the philosophies of Darwin and Sigmund Freud on evolution, debate classmates on the topic of population control, dissect a fetal pig, and perform experiments with flies. However, it also allowed me to skip chemistry and physics, the core of my curriculum as a premed student and chemistry major.

I successfully sold myself on chemistry and physics by telling myself that mathematics, chemistry, physics, and biology were not only just different languages, but also the languages that underlie the very dance of life itself. With this context, I grew to love and excel in fields that had once held dread and fear for me.

In order to heal from pain, we must also create a new context. Instead of seeing pain and suffering as the enemy, the hated, the feared, how can we develop a new context for pain?

"As my sufferings mounted I soon realized that there were two ways in which I could respond to

*my situation – either to react with bitterness or seek
to transform the suffering into a creative force. I
decided to follow the latter course."*
– Martin Luther King Jr.

This quote by Martin Luther King Jr. reminds me of the ancient Tibetan Buddhism practice of tonglen. According to master teacher and best-selling author Pema Chodron: "Tonglen practice, also known as 'taking and sending,' reverses our usual logic of avoiding suffering and seeking pleasure. In tonglen practice, we visualize taking in the pain of others with every in-breath and sending out whatever will benefit them on the out-breath. In the process, we become liberated from age-old patterns of selfishness. We begin to feel love for both ourselves and others; we begin to take care of ourselves and others."

Pema explains that we start by thinking of someone else who is suffering and breathe in with the wish to take all of the pain and suffering away from the person who is suffering. As we breathe out, we send them happiness, joy or whatever they need to feel relief from their suffering. As we do this, we connect with our own fears, anger, pain and suffering ... our own "stuckness." We can then practice using ourselves as the focus, breathing in for ourselves and all others who are also feeling anger, fear, pain and suffering and then breathe out and send compassion for ourselves and all of the other people who are also suffering. Pema goes on to say: "People often say that this practice goes against the grain of how we usually hold ourselves together. Truthfully, this practice does go against the grain of wanting things on our own terms, wanting everything to work out for ourselves no matter what happens to the others. The practice dissolves the walls we've built around our hearts. It dissolves the layers of self-protection we've tried so hard to create. In Buddhist language, one would say that it dissolves the fixation and clinging of ego ... reverses the usual logic of avoiding suffering and seeking pleasure. In the process, we become liberated from very ancient patterns of selfishness. We begin to feel love for both ourselves and others; we begin to take care of ourselves and others." (1)

In a recorded conversation with Pema Chodron, Pulitzer prize winning author and poet Alice Walker refers to this practice from ancient times as a gift passed on to us from our ancestors, who learned to recognize the power of suffering and difficulty as a pathway to wisdom and transformation. If we have the courage to sit with the feeling of sorrow, anger, and suffering rather than run away or escape with all of the usual ways we choose for escape or numb ourselves from the feelings we do not want to have: alcohol, rage, violence, food, sex, overwork, overdoing, shopping, television; somehow, when we choose to sit with our feelings of suffering, pain, fear, anger, they soften our heart. (2)

Similar to the HeartMath study of feelings of anger versus gratitude, we are moving from anger and fear (breakdown physiology), to compassion, and forgiveness of ourselves and others (rest, relax and rebuild physiology). As we breathe in compassion for the suffering of ourselves and others and breathe out hope for ourselves and for all others who are suffering, we will find relief and kindness, which go then will go "with you everywhere, like a shadow or a friend." (From the poem "Kindness" by Naomi Shihab Nye)

I remember the story of a train porter who was featured nationally. Instead of seeing his work as a porter as a scripted monotony, instead of letting others define him, he went to work each day and "sang" the weather to the hundreds of passengers between Connecticut and New York. He loved to sing. He was not a professional singer. He was a porter. But because he had the courage to use his gift (which gave his own daily life more meaning and joy), he brought laughter and enjoyment to hundreds of commuters each day. He was not a professional singer, but he rose to national celebrity because he dared to be true to and listen to his own voice.

Even if we are in a place or job where we know we are not meant to be, by having the courage to be true to ourselves by following our urges, whether it is being true to ourselves where we are, or having the courage to turn in another direction, we will create opportunities which were not previously available and open doors that were not previously open.

In my first year of college, I attended a lecture entitled "How to be Happy." The room was packed, as you might imagine. When the speaker revealed his secret, it seemed so simple, as many secrets are. He said that we usually only celebrate our big accomplishments, graduating from kindergarten, junior high, high school, college, graduate school, getting married, getting our first job, the first promotion, buying our first house. In between these, we struggle to achieve the next big step. We soon forget each single accomplishment as we struggle to achieve the next. We become depressed and angry and fearful and self-deprecating if events occur which we did not have on our "list "of goals or on our list of life's achievements (often set by expectations of our parents, church, the books we have read, the movies we have seen, the lives of others whom we wish to emulate). In this way, between all of the "great achievements," we are caught up in feelings of struggle, pain, suffering, and joylessness. We are on the treadmill. He said that if instead, we learn to congratulate ourselves and appreciate each accomplishment, each encounter, every day, we would find that we would increase our feeling of joy, happiness, well-being, and our feeling of having achieved success.

Pat yourself on the back for waking up (something we frequently don't want to do), making the bed, getting dressed, doing the dishes, getting to work on time, having a successful encounter with a colleague or client, getting through another day, putting one foot in front of the other. We often do these tasks without even thinking, without even taking them in. We "get through" each day, instead of congratulating ourselves and others for all of the courage and skill that it takes to get through every day.

One of the most profound ways of looking at pain and suffering in a new context is again from master Buddhist teacher and one of my favorite authors, Pema Chodron. In her speech to the graduating class of

Naropa University in Boulder, Colorado in the spring of 2014 entitled "Fail, Fail again, Fail Better," she tells the graduates: "I think the most important thing for you kids going out into the world right now is to know how to fail really well." She said that we need to "learn the skill of 'knowing how to hold the pain of things happening that you really don't want to be happening.'" Someone gave me a quote from *Ulysses* where James Joyce writes about how failure can lead to discovery. He actually doesn't use the word *failure*; he uses *errors*, which he says can be "the portals of discovery. It can be hard to tell what's a failure and what's just something that is shifting your life in a different direction. In other words, failure can be the portal to creativity, to learning something new, to having a fresh perspective."

In my own life as an anesthesiologist and pain physician, it is easy to lose perspective and be overcome with fatigue and routine. One of the most important reminders of finding meaning in my life is *The Lost Art of Healing* by eminent Harvard Cardiologist Bernard Lown. As a young cardiologist, he entered the emerging field of interventional cardiology as he felt that it was technology that would lead to the major advances in the diagnosis and treatment of heart disease. After forty years of practice, he writes that he found that it is the simple act of truly listing to patients that holds the most power for healing. In a National Public Radio interview, he gave an example of an interview with a patient who had a history of a severe persistent dysrhythmia, which he had suffered from for eleven years. Dr. Lown told the interviewer that he makes it a practice to interview his patients in his office before they change into the "paper gown," in order to preserve more of their identity as a "person" rather than a "patient." He goes through an extensive history to include past medical history, occupational history, family history and social history. As he asked the gentleman about his family, his wife, and his children, he asked how many grandchildren he had. There was a long pause before the gentleman finally answered. Later, after the patient had changed into his gown, Dr. Lown entered the exam room and was startled to hear the patient say, "Doctor, you cured me!" But, I haven't even examined you," Dr. Lown said to him. "But you have cured me," the patient said again. Then he explained, "When you asked me how many grandchildren I have, I remembered that eleven years ago, my oldest son and I had an argument, a falling out, and he forbade me to ever see his children. I was wondering if I could count them as my grandchildren." After this great loss and sadness came to his awareness, his irregular heartbeat became regular. (4)

Dr. Lown said that indeed, to his surprise, the patient was cured. The irregular heartbeat did not return. He tells many similar stories in his book of the power of patient's fear, anger, extreme sadness, and other emotions to create severe heart disease. And then, he tells of the surprising power of recognition and awareness and "sitting" with these feelings (not running away), to heal the underlying cause of disease. (4)

Just as another renowned Harvard Cardiologist, Dr. Herbert Benson, showed that heart disease could be reversed with mindfulness and awareness practices, his colleague at the Benson-Henry Institute at Massachusetts General Hospital, Dr. John Cabot Zen, found that chronic pain could similarly be reversed. Our awareness and conscious creative use of context can lead to compassion, irony, humor, and surprising twists of fate. As John Lennon put it so very well in the song that he wrote for his son, *Beautiful Boy,* "Life is what happens to you while you're busy making other plans."

Creating Context Exercise:

Sit in a quiet place where you will not be disturbed. If necessary, support your back with pillows so that you are sitting comfortably with your back and neck in a neutral position, feet flat on the floor in front of you, hands resting on your thighs. Observe your breathing, relax your breathing, allow your body to relax, starting at the top of your head and slowly moving down to face, neck, shoulders, arms, hands, back, chest, abdomen, hips, thighs, legs, and feet. Keeping your eyes softly closed, imagine or think of your healing place. Now look at those areas of your life which you are challenged with, but which you are driven and motivated to pursue. Think of the things you love to do and how you can incorporate the spirit of your individual gifts, talents, and personality into the work or challenge that you are facing. How might this pursuit fit in with the other activities, journeys, objectives or dreams of your life? How might it fit in with the attainment of your life goals and aspirations? Quietly sit and slowly observe your breath without actively thinking after asking these questions. If the answer does not come immediately, know that you can come back to the question(s) and that you can continue to "live the question" until you "live into the answer." After the meditation, slowly open your eyes and come back to the present time and place.

Chapter 6

REVERE THE JOURNEY

*"You must live in the present, launch yourself on
every wave, find your eternity in each moment ...
there is no other life but this."*

– Henry David Thoreau

My mother grew up in an American colony
that was established in the State of Sao
Paulo Brazil in the 1800s. She was a
third generation Brazilian and grew up near the small
Brazilian town of Santa Barbara d'Oeste on a sugarcane
plantation. Although she was very proud to become an
American citizen, she always maintained a great love
and identification for the country where she was born,
raised, and educated. She would often share common
Brazilian sayings. "My people, [Brazilians] have lots of
sayings to guide their lives," she would say. So, as to
not let "you Americans" (as she referred to anyone other
than Brazilians, including her children), to be outdone

by "her people," I gathered and collected sayings. One of my favorites has been:

> *"Success is getting what you want. Happiness is*
> *wanting what you get."*
> – Dale Carnegie

I remember one of my medical school classmates, a Harvard graduate whose father was a prominent physician in the town where she grew up. She was following in his footsteps, but by the end of her second year, she made the excruciating and courageous decision to change courses as she realized that this was not her dream nor the road that in her heart, she felt she should follow.

In the modern industrial, scientific, military, political, academic, entertainment, and commercial worlds that we live in, we are steeped in competition, deadlines, resumes, and publish or perish mentalities. There are pervasive cultural, religious, and family tradition-based expectations of what "success" looks like. We prove it to others and to ourselves that we can do what we are "supposed" to do, often at high cost to our health, heart and inner beliefs. Even when we do succeed in what we love to do, we often do not stop, take a breath, exhale, and become aware of the gifts we are given along the way. Life is available only in the *present* moment. We may achieve many successes, but not be able to grasp happiness, as we may not want what we get.

The Physiology of Present Moment Living

"The secret of health for both mind and body is
not to mourn for the past, worry about the future,
or anticipate troubles, but to live in the present
moment wisely and earnestly."
– Buddha

What does this have to do with chronic pain? Although Buddha may not have understood the physiology of pain, he knew from close observation, just as modern system's-based physiology reveals (as we discussed in chapters 2 and 3), that worry, anxiety, fear, and anger are destructive to the mind, emotions, spiritual, and physical aspect of human beings, that constant attachment to the desire for more and more brings about suffering, pain, and ill health. He observed and taught that being present and aware, appreciative of where we are and what we have now in the present moment, is key to the easing of suffering and pain.

Meditation, Mindfulness, and Being Present

When my patients ask about the benefits of meditation and mindfulness and present moment awareness to healing from chronic pain, I tell them that being mindful and paying attention to your breath has more to do with how much pain we have and how we are living our life than they might think. They have the common notion of sitting on the floor, legs crossed, in lotus position with hands in a mudra pose. First of all, I tell them, there are many different types of mindfulness and meditation practices, some sitting, some moving. All, however, use the breath. Deep, slow, relaxed abdominal breathing, in-breaths and slow exhales which are practiced in yogic breathing and mindfulness meditation, stimulate the vagal nerve, which is the command center of the parasympathetic nervous system.

Otto Loewi was awarded a Nobel Prize for his 1921 discovery of *Vagusstof* or vagus stuff (translated into English), later to become known as the neurotransmitter acetylcholine. The vagal nerve controls the parasympathetic nervous system (our rest, relax, and rebuild system). Vagal comes from the Latin root vagus which means wandering. The vagal nerve is the longest nerve in the body. It "wanders" from the brain throughout the body to all of the internal organs, sense organs, blood vessels, and to a portion of skin of the outer ear.

GABA is another neural chemical or neurotransmitter released by the vagal nerve. Yogic breathing has been shown to increase the neurotransmitter GABA, which is deficient in individuals with anxiety, depression, and post-traumatic stress disorder. Recent studies have shown that yogic breathing and mindfulness practice can increase heart rate variability (associated with longevity, health, and youth), coherence of heart, lungs, and brain, and improve mood. (1, 2)

Here again is the correlation seen with modern quantum physics and quantum biology. We cannot separate mental, physical, and spiritual aspects of who we are. So, when we exhale mindfully, we are letting go of all that is no longer needed at physical, mental, and spiritual levels. We are letting go, at the physical level, of toxins and tension that we have been holding onto that are no longer useful. We are letting go of mental tension and toxic thoughts that are no longer useful, and letting go of hopelessness, joylessness, and suffering that are no longer serving us. This makes room for inhaling a new breath, one that has everything that we need on the physical level for health and life. At the mental and emotional level, with the inhale we may realize that we have everything around us that we need to support us in this moment. At the level of spirit, with the inhale we take in all that is necessary to be present in this moment and be aware of all that is available at the level of spirit … from ourselves, the earth, and others, to live our lives.

The Secret to Healthy Digestion and Decreasing Pain

As part of my study of Integrative Medicine and Holistic systems, I studied Ayurvedic medicine concepts. It is taught in ancient Ayurvedic teachings, that if one has "Agni," or a hot digestive fire, then you could even eat, not the healthiest diet, but would be able to extract or metabolize, "burn" up, and extract all of the life force from the food. Whereas someone who does not have a hot digestive fire could eat the healthiest food, but the food would not be utilized or metabolized, but would create toxic residue, like a substance that is smoldering and giving off toxic smoke and gas. What makes us have a "hot" digestive fire, I asked myself.? Of course, the vagal nerve and the parasympathetic nervous system!

Since we activate and train the vagal nerve and the parasympathetic nervous system when we meditate or practice mindfulness, we are building our "Agni" or hot digestive fire. When we slowly, mindfully eat, we are breaking down the food and mixing it with the many enzymes contained in our saliva and protective proteins which help it to be better absorbed and broken down in the stomach and intestines. We produce the pancreatic enzymes and optimize the motility or movement of our digestive system so that we fully absorb nutrients and fully let go of and eliminate toxic wastes. When we stimulate the vagal nerve, we are decreasing cortisol, increasing metabolism (shedding unwanted fat and weight), and decreasing inflammation. When we eat mindfully, we also take in the colors, smells, and tastes of the food, which further stimulates optimal digestion along with a state of emotional well-being. We are also turning down the sympathetic nervous system, the break down mode, and turning on the parasympathetic nervous system, the body's relax, digest, and assimilate, rebuild mode, which helps us to heal from injury and from chronic pain.

As we practice awareness with eating, breathing, and walking, we become more aware of ourselves, who we are, and who we are compatible with. We see and hear things around us that we had never seen or appreciated before (when we were walking while texting or catching up on email or fitting in a conference call on the way to our next meeting or on our way home, were in our head rehearsing worry and fear instead of looking at the surrounding beauty). Instead of stuffing our feelings and thoughts undigested into some compartment to deal with "later" when we find some "free" time, we can take this very moment to truly be aware of and "digest and assimilate" our lives.

Mary Burmeister, who brought the Art of Jin Shin Jyutsu, an ancient Japanese healing art form, from Japan to the United States and spread it throughout the world, said, "In ignorance one specializes in parts, in wisdom one focuses on the whole." I am especially drawn to this ancient healing art form because of its emphasis on self-help and self-efficacy. Mary Burmeister taught that, "The truth is that within each one of us lies the power to cast all misery aside and to KNOW complete Peace and Oneness – to be that beautiful creation of perfect harmony - to truly KNOW (help) MYSELF."

Mary studied the art of Jin Shin Jyutsu for many years with Master Jiro Murai, a philosopher and son in a long line of physicians, born the late 1800s in Japan. Master Murai studied the Bible, ancient Greek, Indian, Chinese, and Japanese texts. He rediscovered this lost art, which had been passed down through generations, an innate art of mankind with origins from before Moses, before Gautama Buddha. In Jin Shin Jyutsu, the hands are used as "jumper cables" to harmonize the breath, one's awareness, and the function and energy of the mind body and spirit. Mary taught that Jin Shin Jyutsu means "The art of the Creator through compassionate man" in Japanese. "Physio-philosophy" that is used by everyone unconsciously, doesn't "do" anything, yet encompasses everything. "I call it the art of life, the art of life itself." She said that, "As we abuse our bodies in our daily routines, mentally, emotionally, digestively, or physically, our safety energy locking system becomes activated … this is simply to let us know we are abusing our bodies." Using light touch, we can unlock or free areas of blockage or tension in the body, mind, and spirit, which may present as pain, suffering, or attitudes. (3)

In Jin Shin Jyutsu, each organ function energy is associated with physical, mental, emotional, and spiritual attributes which present differently based on the level of harmony or disharmony of the body. For example, the large intestine function energy becomes stomach function energy at eight a.m. and flows from the cheek bone up to the center between the eyebrows, crosses to under the opposite eye, descends to and follows the jawbone line up to the front to the opposite ear above eyebrow line, turns toward the eyes, and descends down the front of the face and neck to the acromion under the collar bone where it divides into parts A and B. A and B parts of the stomach function energy flow travel to the umbilicus or navel, to the spleen, kidneys, gall bladder, twelfth thoracic vertebra, to the medial and outer thighs, knees, outer leg, top of foot, and first three toes. (3)

As observed by Master Murai over a lifetime dedicated to the study of the art of Jin Shin Jyutsu, disharmony of each organ function can be observed as tension or asymmetries involving the organ function energy path in the physical body, in disharmony in emotions associated with that organ function energy, or with disharmony in the spiritual aspects associated with that organ function energy. He observed that disharmony of stomach function energy from overload could result in depression or insanity (at the mental and emotional levels) and on the physical level, hot perspiring skin surface, a bloody or stuffy nose, dry mouth and chapped lips, dark complexion, swelling of neck, numbness of throat, abdominal bloating, pain and swelling of the knee cap, stiff middle finger, discomfort above breast, appendix, abdomen, groin, inner ankle, and top of instep. He also gave examples of deficiency of stomach function energy that could be observed as goose flesh appearing over the body, stomach feeling cold and chilly, and abdomen bloating. (3)

The practitioner of Jin Shin Jyutsu in addition to "listening" to the pulses, observes or "reads" the body. Each "organ function energy" flows throughout the body in a certain pattern (similar to acupuncture meridians) and may affect many aspects of the body, mind, and spiritual function of the human being. By looking at the body, listening to the voice, the words (for attitudes of anger, sadness, fear, worry, or pretense), and then, gently holding or touching fingers, toes, and body areas in simple sequences, harmony can be restored. But, as Mary would say, "The physical, mental, and emotional may be cleaned up for now, but if we go out and dirty it up again, we need to clean up the dirt, dust, and grime again. That's all it is. You'll just come in for more housecleaning, or you'll do it yourself."(3)

In addition to using the flows, breath and awareness, Jin Shin Jyutsu students are taught that it is an art and not a technique and that each moment, and each day, we can practice living the art of Jin Shin Jyutsu.

A simple but profound Jin Shin Jyutsu treatment is to hold our fingers. The energy pathways flow through the fingers and toes. The fingers are usually more accessible than our toes, so by simply wrapping the fingers and thumb of the opposite hand gently around a thumb or finger of the opposite hand, we are using our "jumper cable" energy to harmonize that energy pathway. For example, to harmonize stomach and spleen organ function energy, simply wrap the fingers and thumb of your right hand gently around the left thumb. Babies and small children suck their thumbs to self-sooth, to help them sleep, to help with digestion. We can also self-soothe, help ourselves fall asleep, help with digestion, help to let go of excess worry. By gently holding our thumb for even two to three minutes we will feel a calm, more grounded feeling. Holding the index finger helps with neck and back tension and to release excess fear. Holding the middle finger helps to let go of excess anger and frustration and helps to harmonize liver and gall bladder function energy. Gently holding onto the ring finger helps to harmonize lung and large intestine function energy, helps us to breath more easily and helps us to let go of excess sadness. Finally, gently holding the little finger helps us to let go of "pretense," of smiling on the outside and crying on the inside, trying too hard … a life of too much effort. The art of Jin Shin Jyutsu teaches us, as Mary said, to become a "Human Being," not a "Human Trying to Be." (3)

Making Space

Becoming aware can help you to realize the impact that your environment is having on your well-being.

Your home and workplace spaces can either nurture and support your well-being or deplete you and leave you feeling chaotic. "The impact architecture has on a person's mood is huge. Arguably these are the fundamentals of architecture: not how it looks, but how we feel it, through the way it allows us to act, behave, think, and reflect," says Dr. Melanie Dodd, program director of spatial practices at the Central St Martins art school.

We may not be able to rebuild the structure of our home and work environments; however, we can take time to clear out clutter and items that bring up feelings of anxiety and toxic memories. This can also decrease the chaos of looking for lost keys, books, or papers, for example. Decluttering can create a calm and peaceful space that allows you to relax and regenerate. We can also then begin to add items that remind us of meaningful and fun experiences and pictures of people who elevate and encourage us.

Become aware of how different colors affect you. Color impacts mood, appetite, energy level and body temperature. Learn to use color and nurturing plants, natural lighting, and other natural elements to enhance your feelings of well-being at your home and work spaces. According to Walch et al, 2005, rooms with brighter natural and artificial lights caused spine surgery patients to take less pain medication and experience less pain. Studies also report that incorporating natural elements or scenes of nature may have positive effects on mood in both healthy and depressed individuals. (4)

Simple Things

Two of my favorite poems remind me to take pleasure in the simple pleasures and gifts that surround us every day, those things we often overlook and take for granted. The first is "Ode To my Socks" from the collection of poems entitled *Ode to Common Things* by Pablo Neruda. The other poem is by former US Poet Laureate Billy Collins in his collection *Nine Horses*, entitled "Aimless Love." I encourage you to find and read these poems as they teach us how simple rituals can become a journey of discovery; putting on your socks, washing your hands, smelling the soap, the rain, watching the cat on the fence, and listening to the birds can become treasured rituals. We can create a life filled with gratitude and awareness; – a life with no ordinary moments.

Meaning in the Randomness

I often mention in my lectures, "the best book that I never read." I was at the bookstore, reading flap covers of books on the discounted display. I read a few as I walked by, then later, an idea from the flap cover of one of the books kept coming back to me. The book was called, *God's Invitation List*. It suggested the possibility that all of the people that we meet, in the elevator, in the store, at work, are perhaps not randomly crossing our paths, but are on "God's invitation list" to our lives. This thought has made me much more mindful of the people I cross paths with throughout my days. Perhaps we most reflect who we are when we interact with those whom we believe have no impact on the outcome of our lives. In the same way, I have had some of the most meaningful conversations, learned great wisdom, and have heard stories of great courage from conversations with strangers on a plane or a train or in a waiting room. This perhaps is digesting the light or spiritual aspects of life. We can exhale and let go of the past and make room to breathe in and become aware of and assimilate the beauty and courage and strength of living creatures, nature, and other human beings.

The difficulty of being in the present moment is to not fear or worry, but to have the courage to live with uncertainty. There is so much that we don't know, but perhaps there is a way to live with patience, curiosity and awe at the questions themselves. As beloved poet Reiner Maria Rilke said:

> *"Be patient toward all that is unsolved in your heart-try to love the questions themselves like locked rooms and like books that are written in a very foreign tongue. Do not now seed the answers, which cannot be given you because you would not be able to live them. And the point is, to live everything. Live the questions now. Perhaps you will then gradually, without noticing it, live along some distant day into the answer."*
>
> – Rilke

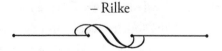

Exercise: Creating Inner Spaciousness

We can create inner stillness, spaciousness, and stability using meditation and visualization. A powerful and well-known meditation taught by Vietnamese

Buddhist monk Thich Nhat Hanh is called the four-pebble meditation. We begin by placing four pebbles in our left hand. Take the first pebble from the left hand and place it in the right hand while visualizing a fresh flower. Think to yourself that we are each flowers in the garden of humanity. When we are young, our skin is fresh, our thoughts are fresh, our eyes are fresh, and our smiles are fresh. As we grow old we can lose that freshness. However, we can become fresh again with new thoughts, fresh hopes, fresh dreams, and fresh lives. Think with the in breath, "I am a flower," and with the out breath, "I am fresh." With three breaths, say on each in breath, "flower" and on each out breath, "Fresh.

Now take the second pebble from the left hand to the right and think of a mountain that is strong and solid. Think of feeling the inner strength and stability of a mountain, stable and strong for you and others. Take three breaths. With each in breath say "Mountain," with each out breath say to yourself, "Solid."

Now move the third pebble from the left hand to the right hand. Think of a clear mountain lake that reflects things as they truly are, unlike turbulent or raging water, which distorts images. Take three breaths. On the in breath say to yourself, "Clear water," on the out breaths say silently to yourself, "true reflection."

Finally, take the fourth pebble and as you transfer the pebble from your left hand to your right hand, think of space, the sky, spaciousness, and the free feeling associated with this spaciousness. Take three breaths. With each in breath say silently to yourself, "Space," and with each out breath, "Free."

PART THREE

Chapter 7

YOU ARE NOT YOUR MRI

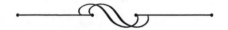

"Our Knowledge of the elementary grammar of the world continues to grow. If we try to put together what we have learned about the physical world in the course of the twentieth century, the clues point toward something profoundly different from what we were taught in school. An elementary structure of the world is emerging generated by a swarm of quantum events where time and space do not exist. Quantum fields draw together space, time, matter and light, exchanging information between one event and another. Reality is a network of granular events; the dynamic that connects them is probabilistic; between one event and another, space, time, matter, and energy melt into a cloud of probability."
– Italian Physicist Carlo Rovelli

A few years ago, at a medical acupuncture training, a colleague of mine was discussing his chronic low back pain with the instructor of the course, a renowned sports medicine physician from McGill University in Canada whose patients included elite Olympic and professional athletes and professional dancers. The professor asked my colleague about his low back pain, and my friend proceeded to demonstrate his pain with limited forward and backward bending of his lumbar spine, and pain with turning from side to side. He told the professor that his MRI showed significant degeneration of the disc at the L4-5 and L5-S1 levels. During the five-day course, the sports medicine physician proceeded to treat my colleague. After three treatments, he was able to bend forward, touch his toes, turn from side to side and bend backward with much greater range of motion, with no pain. He has continued to receive acupuncture and has also begun to meditate and initiate other healthy lifestyle practices.

Of course, his MRI did not change over the five-day course. So then, how could his pain improve and his MRI be the same? This is very confusing to most individuals, because our materialistic view of reality is such that we believe that we are like a table or a car, which once broken, cannot get better unless it is "fixed" by a specialist. If we cannot see something, we do not understand how it can exist. We do not understand the new vision of reality understood by quantum physicists, that at our core, at the level of our subatomic structure, "Quantum fields draw together space, time, matter and light, exchanging information between one event and another. Reality is a network of granular events; the dynamic that connects them is probabilistic; between one event and another, space, time, matter, and energy melt into a cloud of probability." Carlo Rovelli

It's Not Either-Or

My focus on non-interventional and non-pharmacologic methods of pain management may have led you to believe that I do not believe in or support conventional Western medical modalities of treatment. In fact, my day to-day practice consists of evaluating patients in a conventional Western pain management practice where we evaluate and care for patients with a wide variety of complaints.

Many of my patients have low back pain (the number one pain complaint of Western industrialized nations), neck pain, and headaches. We also see patients who have persistent pain after various types of surgeries, following non-surgical injuries such as sprains after which their pain has lingered, patients with widespread pain and patients with pain due to cancer, or patients with common or rare diseases where chronic pain is but one component or part of the disease.

In many cases our patients come to us suffering from chronic severe unremitting pain. Many of these patients also have co-existing depression, anxiety, post-traumatic stress disorder, insomnia, and mental health disorders. Although our goal is always to help the patient to return to a state of health and well-being, we do realize that this may take some time. As such, we offer the safest and most effective medications combined with non-medication modalities (topical medications, transcutaneous, electrical stimulation units, physical medicine and rehabilitation, wellness modalities such as mindfulness training, yoga, Qigong, Tai Chi, nutritional education) and appropriate interventional pain injections such as epidural steroid injections, trigger point injections to relieve persistent muscle spasm, radiofrequency ablation to alleviate pain associated with arthritis of facet joints of the spine and even advanced procedures such as non-surgical electro thermal disc treatment and implantation of spinal cord stimulators for patients with intractable nerve related pain. We also perform regenerative medicine procedures such as injection of platelet-rich plasma and other approved cutting-edge stem cell promoting medical products that promote and accelerate healing of musculoskeletal injuries. For patients with neuropathic pain, we can administer infusions of ketamine, lidocaine, or magnesium, which are helpful in many patients. In addition, if a patient's history or examination combined with imaging studies reveals a need for surgical treatment, we not infrequently consult our surgical colleagues and refer our patients to them for further evaluation. We also work closely with and refer our patients frequently to psychiatrists and health psychologists who evaluate and treat the mental health of our patients.

Our patients often have significant relief following the above therapies, but a frequent question which they pose is, "Will I have to take these medications and have to suffer with side effects of the medications for the rest of my life?" or "Will I continue to get worse and need surgery?" or " … will I need another surgery." So, I then begin to tell them about the scientific evidence of how changing our lifestyle choices can harmonize the underlying systems such as the immune system, autonomic nervous system, and neuroendocrine systems to allow the body to repair itself, to improve our health our well-being and our pain.

One of the most difficult concepts for our patients to grasp is the concept of frequent lack of correlation between pain and x-rays and Magnetic Resonance Imaging (MRI) findings. It can be extremely frustrating for patients to have severe back pain and pain radiating into their leg or legs, or in their neck and radiating into their arms and hands and have minimal degenerative disc changes, or changes on their MRI which do not correspond in location or severity to their presenting symptoms. Many patients with severe back and neck pain have a complete lack of degenerative disc findings on their MRI!

The opposite also occurs, in that patients with minimal or no pain will have images that show severe degenerative disc disease and nerve compression. I have had discussions with my neurosurgeon colleagues regarding MRIs of patients who initially present with large disc bulges on their spine MRIs, who choose to not have surgery and on follow up, either with the spine surgeon or with the pain clinic, have new MRIs showing resolution of the disc bulge within periods ranging from six months to three years. I cannot find any prospective studies looking at factors associated with improvement versus worsening of degenerative disc disease, but perhaps, as our medical system continues to adopt a preventive approach, and as we become more familiar as a society with the idea that our health and biologic age can improve as we age chronologically, instead of worsening, more studies examining the question of how we can best heal ourselves will be performed.

The correlation between back pain and the presence of degenerative disc and spine changes on x-rays and MRIs is a complex and controversial area of study. In general, it is known that whether or not we develop back pain, by the time we are in our mid 60s, more than 94% of us will have MRI and x-ray findings showing degenerative changes of the spine.

There are numerous studies which show no correlation between current back pain and degenerative disc findings on MRI, and others which do find a correlation between degenerative discs on MRI and low back pain. This may be because some individuals have constant low back pain, while others have low back pain which is intermittent or which comes and goes, however, current studies in patients with no low back pain but a history of low back pain, show that degenerative disc disease does not predict future back pain. (1, 2)

Back and neck pain can also be associated with structures other than the discs which lie between the vertebra of the spine. Back pain can be associated with arthritis of the joints in the back of the spine known as facet joints, with the many ligaments of the spine, and/or with the many large muscles located along the side of the spine. Diagnosis of the source of back pain can be difficult and require multiple diagnostic and therapeutic trials, as the pain referral pattern associated with each of these structures is similar, due to overlap of the nerves supplying the discs, facet joints, and muscles at each level.

Stress, anxiety, chronic insomnia, depression, and chronic fatigue may also contribute to chronic or recurrent pain as each of these increases sympathetic activity (remember that pain fibers are part of the sympathetic nervous system/fight or flight or adrenalin system, so stress can activate pain), cortisol levels, and inflammation. In addition, there are the "software" changes or up regulation of the pain in the spinal cord and areas of the brain which process pain and these "neuroplastic changes" occur over time in individuals with persistent or large-scale pain signaling.

The presence of these additional stress and mental health disorders vary across the population of individuals with low back pain. It has been shown that anxiety, depression, and poorly controlled chronic disease are individual risk factors associated with the development of chronic pain after surgery. Thus, these individuals may be less likely to obtain relief of pain following surgery. A multidisciplinary approach (including psychologic, psychiatric, rehabilitative approaches) is recommended in these individuals with "complex pain," to address the mental, psychological and emotional components which are contributing to their pain.

Even so, studies report that those individuals who remain passive and believe that they have no personal control over their pain are more likely to continue to suffer from chronic pain compared to those individuals who become active participants in their health care. Indeed, a recent study of more than 12,000 men and

10,000 women in Scandinavia showed that a healthy lifestyle (defined as a combination of non-smoking, no-risk consumption of alcohol, recommended level of leisure physical activity and recommended consumption of fruit and vegetables) is associated with a decrease in the risk of developing troublesome back pain over a period of four years among individuals with occasional low back pain and neck pain. (3)

> *"The natural healing force within each of us is the greatest force in getting well."*
> – Hippocrates

An anesthesiologist and pain management physician colleague, after travel to Vietnam on a humanitarian mission a few years ago, related his experience in a conference upon his return. On the mission, the surgical and medical teams, in addition to performing much needed surgeries and providing other medical care, met a Vietnamese physician. My colleague told us that this Vietnamese physician changed his view on integrative medicine approaches. She told him that because there was very little access to modern medical and surgical techniques by much of the population there in Vietnam, there was a strong reliance on preventive medicine approaches and complementary and alternative approaches and helping the body to heal by non-surgical and non-pharmacologic means.

Here in the United States and in much of the Western industrial nations, because we have access to such highly-developed medical and surgical technology and pharmacologic therapies, we have, like the space ship humans in the movie *Wally*, become less self-sufficient and see ourselves, as Descartes and the other scientists of the 1400s to 1700s did, as a clock whose parts can be "fixed" or "replaced" by others. If we think of the opening of the arteries of the heart at one and five years in the Dr. Dean Ornish study of severe heart disease patients who made healthy lifestyle changes, compared to worsening of heart disease in similar patients who had the best of modern surgery, angioplasty. and medication but who did not make healthy lifestyle changes; if we remember Dr. Art Bernstein who continued to have severe back pain after three surgeries but was able get off medications and return to surfing and a normal life after adopting healthy lifestyle changes, we can see that we do not have to define ourselves by what we see on the x-ray, CT scan or MRI.

My hope is that we can begin to educate our children and ourselves as to the much more immense possibilities that we have as human beings, for self-care, and self-healing. By this I do not mean that we should abandon the wonders of modern technology. I do not think that it is an either-or choice. As Italian physicist Carlo Rovelli wrote in his 2016 book, *Reality is Not What It Seems:*

> *"Scientific thinking explores and redraws the world,
> gradually offering us better and better images
> of it, teaching us to think in ever more effective
> ways. Science is a continual exploration of ways
> of thinking. Its strength is its visionary capacity to
> demolish preconceived ideas, to reveal new regions*

of reality and to construct new and more effective images of the world. This adventure rests upon the entirety of past knowledge but at its heart is change. The world is boundless and iridescent; we want to go and see it. We are immersed in its mystery and in its beauty, and over the horizon there is unexplored territory. The incompleteness and uncertainty of our knowledge, our precariousness suspended over the abyss of the immensity of what we don't know, does not render life meaningless, it makes it interesting and precious."

– Carlo Rovelli

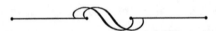

Exercise: The Only Thing That Is Constant Is Change

Sit in a quiet place where you will not be disturbed. If necessary, support your back with pillows so that you are sitting comfortably with your back and neck in a neutral position, feet flat on the floor in front of you, hands resting on your thighs. Observe your breathing, relax your breathing, allow your abdomen to relax and expand as you inhale and very naturally fall back as you exhale. Shift your focus softly to your left big toe. Feel the sensation of your toe inside your shoe or on the floor. Sense the top, bottom, sides, and tip of your big toe. Now shift your attention to any thoughts which are bubbling up in your mind, gently observe them non-judgmentally and let them go with your exhale. Now slowly turn your attention to your right fifth finger, as it relaxes on your thigh. Feel the back, front, base, and tip of your right fifth finger … the temperature of the air, any small breezes, or just the feeling of the air as it surrounds your finger. Now shift your attention back to your left first toe. Note any sameness or differences in how you are now sensing or feeling your toe, your finger, and your body. You can continue this exercise for fifteen to twenty minutes and just observe various parts of your body, the sensation of the space around you. If thoughts bubble up, return your attention to your breath. Finally feel the sense of your entire body, thoughts, feelings, and your connection to the space surrounding you. Imagine yourself sitting on a boat, which is floating slowly down the clear blue river. Now you feel as if you are weightless, with the strange sensation that you are now both sitting in the boat on the river and looking down at the river as it curls though the fields, valleys, and hills. Now you have a sense of journey, of where you have been and where you are going as you see the winding river from this view. Now you feel your awareness returning to the boat. The moment now seems timeless as you drift slowly down the river. It feels as if the moment will last forever. You have no sensation of where you have been or where you are going. You are aware only of this moment. Relax into this feeling, then slowly, when you are ready, open your eyes and return to the present moment.

Chapter 8

DIET AND VITAMIN D

*"The doctor of the future will give no medication
but will interest his patients in the care of the
human frame, diet and in the cause and prevention
of disease."*
– Thomas Edison

In 2010, I attended for the first time, an annual conference held by the Scripps Center for Integrative Medicine in La Jolla entitled *Natural Supplements: An Evidence-based Update*. Speakers included the leading investigators from the National Institute of Health and other leading scientists and clinicians in the field of Integrative Medicine. The audience consisted of hundreds of medical and osteopathic physicians and surgeons and other allied health care specialists and providers. During one of the panel discussions, a fit, white-haired physician stood up at one of the microphones placed for the audience to ask questions of the panelists. He paused, looked at the panelists and around at the audience and said: "In the 1960s, I attended UCLA medical school. During my four years of medical school, we had one hour of education on nutrition in my first year of medical school. My grandson is now attending UCLA medical school, one of the best medical schools in the country, and he received one hour of education on nutrition in his first year of medical school."

The point that he was making was that we as physicians are educated primarily to treat patients using a disease management approach, and not a health promoting and preventive approach. Although the evidence being presented to us at this conference on the health benefits of various nutrients and supplements was based on rigorous research which had been published in peer reviewed medical journals, the majority of the audience, many of us who were one or more decades into our professional practices, were hearing it for the first time.

I was most impressed by the evidence presented on vitamin D. First of all, I was not aware that vitamin D guidelines were published by the Society of Endocrinology, the medical specialty that diagnoses and manages diseases such as diabetes, which are associated with hormone imbalances. This is because vitamin D is considered a pro hormone. I was not aware that vitamin D deficiency and insufficiency is associated with low back pain and wide spread pain, or that there is a worldwide pandemic of vitamin D deficiency, even in children and adolescents. This is because vitamin D is found in very few foods, making it very difficult to obtain adequate levels from food sources. Additionally, vitamin D absorbed from sunlight must undergo complex enzymatic changes in the liver and the kidney and vitamin D from food sources must be adequately taken up in the stomach and intestine. There are many factors that affect the body's ability to make and absorb vitamin D. These factors include: where you live, the season, how much time you spend outdoors without sunscreen, genetic variability, skin pigmentation, age, obesity, pollution, having healthy intestines with optimal absorption capacity, and various medications which may interfere with absorption.

I was not aware that vitamin D has steroid-like effects in the whole body and regulates the expression of more than one hundred genes by way of vitamin D receptor (VDR). Many studies have shown that vitamin D has multiple protective effects on the nervous system. Among these is the regulation of nerve growth factor (NGF), which is responsible for the development of new neurons, and for the health and maintenance of mature ones. It is also an antioxidant that controls the process of detoxification in the brain and nervous system. (1)

According to NIH-funded scientists David Feldman MD and Peter J. Malloy PhD in their 2010 article, *Genetic Disorders and Defects in Vitamin D action*, "In recent years there have been many new actions attributed to vitamin D that mediate important and wide-spread effects that are unrelated to calcium and bone homeostasis. These include actions to reduce the risk of cancer, autoimmune disease, infection, neurodegeneration, etc." (2)

Recent observational and prospective studies suggest that vitamin D may play a significant role in preventing respiratory infections, cardiovascular health, cancer, autoimmune disease such as multiple sclerosis and type one diabetes and, in pregnancy, prevention of pregnancy related diabetes, preeclampsia, and premature birth. (3)

According to the National Institutes of Health, vitamin D, in addition to promoting calcium absorption in the gut, maintaining blood calcium and phosphate levels needed for bone heath and growth, and prevention of osteoporosis in older adults, is also important in the regulation of cell growth, differentiation, and cell turnover. It also is important in neuromuscular function and reduction of inflammation. (4)

Although the inactive source of vitamin D can be obtained from sunlight, is not recommended that we increase our exposure to sunlight and other sources of UV light as this increases our risk of skin cancer. Additionally, it is known that some individuals and families are not able to effectively convert the inactive form of vitamin D into the active form of vitamin D. This complex conversion requires enzymatic steps in the liver and in the kidney. It is also very difficult to obtain adequate amounts of vitamin D from food sources. Because of this, supplementation with the active form of vitamin D, vitamin D3 has been recommended.

Due to the large amount of evidence regarding the importance of vitamin D in both musculoskeletal and many non-musculoskeletal health functions, the Society of Endocrinology published new guidelines in 2011 recommending 400-600 IU/day for zero to one year and one to eighteen-year-old children and adolescents for musculoskeletal health while stating that "However, to raise the blood level of 25(OH)D (Vitamin D) consistently above 30 ng/ml ... [low normal level of vitamin d] may require at least 1000 IU/d of vitamin."

For adults, the minimum daily requirement for musculoskeletal health was raised to 600 IU -800IU/day for 70-70+ adults, with the caveat, "It is unknown whether 600 IU/d is enough to provide all the potential nonskeletal health benefits associated with vitamin D. However, to raise the blood level of 25(OH)D consistently above 30 ng/ml may require at least 1500 – 2000 IU/d of vitamin D3." (5)

For patients with chronic low back pain or wide spread pain, a baseline vitamin D level is recommended. I recommend that my adult patients take 1500 to 2000 IU/day, as is recommended by the guidelines of the society of endocrinology to maintain levels between 30 (low normal) and 75 ng/ml. (5) For pregnant women, 4,000 IU/day of vitamin D3 is now recommended. (6)

Although this book is not meant to be a comprehensive guide to nutrition, nutrition is an important component of overall health and thus for healing from injury and chronic pain. I do recommend, however, that a healthy diet be combined with the mindfulness and stress reduction practices that I have discussed in previous chapters, as even the best food will not be digested, assimilated, and distributed to where it is needed in the body in someone who is in the chronic stress/sympathetic nervous system/adrenalin/fight or flight mode.

In general, healthy diet recommendations are fairly simple. They include eating a variety of vegetables of all types – dark green, red, orange, beans, peas, starchy vegetables, fruits (whole fruits are the healthiest option), whole grains, a variety of protein foods including seafood, lean meat, and poultry, eggs, beans, peas, nuts, seeds and soy produces, and healthy oils such as extra virgin olive oil. We should limit or avoid processed foods. In addition to containing often unhealthy additives and dyes, processed foods do not contain the protective phytochemical and other important health-promoting benefits of whole foods. Healthy eating also includes consuming less than 10% of daily calories from added sugars, avoiding or limiting processed or artificial sugars (good choices are natural sugars such as maple syrup), limiting calories from saturated fats to less than 10% of calories consumed per day, and consuming less than 2,300 milligrams per day of sodium.

If alcohol is consumed, it should be consumed in moderation – up to one drink per day for women and up to two drinks per day for men – and only by adults of legal drinking age. (7)

Of course, individuals should speak with their doctors or dietitians before making any changes to their diets.

What you eat, interestingly, is only part of the story. Longevity and health is most significantly affected by how much we eat. At the conference that I attended in 2010, scientists reported that after initial research on mice showed dramatic improvements in overall health and longevity following restriction of calories, a similar experiment was performed on Rhesus monkey liter mates. The monkey who was given the 30% caloric restricted diet starting at age sixteen (the equivalent of middle age in humans), at age twenty-two, when photographed side by side with his litter mate who was allowed to eat as much as he liked, looked young, sleek, and muscular, while his litter mate who did not have caloric restriction was not only heavier, but looked many years older, like the grandfather of the caloric restricted monkey. According to an article published in *Scientific American* in February 2016, the caloric restricted monkey "is now 43, a longevity record for the species, according to the study, and the equivalent of a human living to 130." In addition to longevity benefits, cancer and cardiovascular disease in calorie-restricted monkeys is about 50% reduced.

Biochemist Valter Longo, a professor of biologic science at USC who runs the Longevity Institute at the USC Leonard Davis School of Letters, Arts, and Sciences, states that "though a diet rich in vegetables, legumes, fish, nuts and whole grains, can provide the least costly way to take care of a lot of problems and can be key to a longer and healthier life," periodic fat mimicking diets (five days a month of a low-protein, low sugar, and relatively high fat diet for three months in a recent prospective randomized crossover study in human subjects), have shown benefits which include reduced body weight, body fat, lowered blood pressure, decreased IGF-1 (which is implicated in aging and disease), decreased cholesterol, triglycerides, blood glucose and c-reactive protein (a marker of inflammation).

Per the scientists who conducted the study, "Larger studies in patients with diagnosed diseases or selected on the basis of risk factors are warranted to confirm the effect of the Fasting mimicking diet on disease prevention and treatment." (8)

According to Dr. Longo, studies show that long-lived populations around the world eat a diet that is mostly plant-based, low in protein, and rich in unsaturated fats and complex carbohydrates. The science shows that it is very important to stick to twelve hours of eating and twelve hours of fasting during each day. Eating fifteen or more hours per day "starts to be associated with metabolic problems, sleep disorders, etc." while fasting for longer than twelve to thirteen hours per day can be associated with "problems like gallstone formation." He states that data also shows that skipping breakfast is associated with increased risk of cardiovascular disease and overall mortality.

Interestingly, caloric sparing means the opposite of going hungry. It means eating the right food combinations in the right amounts which signal to your stomach and your brain that you are full. Dr. Longo gives an example of "two ounces of pasta with seven ounces of garbanzo beans, four ounces of vegetables and about three tablespoons of olive oil. This gives you a good amount of protein, provides a lot of vitamins and minerals, keeps the simple carbohydrates to a limited amount and fills your stomach." (9)

For great healthy recipes using healthy ingredients, Dr. Andrew Weil has recently published a new book entitled *Fast Food, Good Food: More Than 150 Quick and Easy Ways to Put Healthy, Delicious Food on the Table.* There are also many other excellent free online sources of recipes for Mediterranean diet/anti-inflammatory diet. (10)

Water for Relief and Healing from Pain

As an anesthesiologist and from my study of biochemistry as an undergraduate in college, I realize the importance of adequate hydration to decrease pain and optimize the digestion, assimilation, and elimination of our food. Our body is approximately 70% water. At the basic molecular level, water is involved in processes such as hydrolysis, where water reacts with a chemical to break it into smaller molecules. Many chemical reactions occur in our cells. Together these are referred to "metabolism." Each chemical involved is called a "metabolite." Water is a reactant or is a product or result of a reaction.

In addition to being involved in cellular metabolism, water is essential for temperature regulation. Our enzymes, which catalyze (cause or accelerate a process) many chemical reactions in the body, operate within a very narrow range of temperature. Water acts to buffer temperature changes in the body because of its relatively high specific heat capacity (the heat required to raise one kilogram of water by one degree centigrade), its relatively large enthalpy of vaporization (heat energy required to convert a liquid to a gas), and enthalpy of fusion (energy required to convert a solid to a liquid), as reflected in water's relatively high boiling and melting points. Also, many chemicals dissolve in water and so it acts as a transporter of these molecules in and out of the cells. Water is also important in bonding and ion exchange, as well as in the structure and function of proteins, nucleic acids, and other components of cellular structure and function. (11)

At the level of delivery of oxygen and nutrients to the body, if we are chronically dehydrated, our body's survival mechanisms kick in. It will minimize the blood sent to the musculoskeletal parts of the body in order to perfuse or supply the brain and vital organs (heart, kidneys, liver, spleen, intestines, lungs) with blood. Think of the heart as a pump. There is the fluid (blood, in the case of the body) coming to the heart, the rate of the pump (our heart rate), the pump engine (the muscles of the heart involved in contraction and ejection or pumping of the blood out to the body, and the "afterload" which is the pressure which the left ventricle of the heart must overcome to get blood to the body. Constriction or resistance of the peripheral arteries is part of the afterload equation.

If we are dehydrated, we have a decrease in preload or blood coming to the heart, so the body compensates by increasing the heart rate, increasing the force of the heart muscle to pump what blood there is with increased pressure to the vital parts of the body, and lastly, it increases peripheral constriction of the vessels which supply the musculoskeletal system (in order to have the pressure to supply the brain and vital organs with the reduced volume).

Since water is needed to hydrate mucinous proteins which act as lubricants and protectants for the joints and tissues as they slide over each other during movement, with dehydration, we have more chance of breakdown due to lack of nutrients and oxygen for normal cellular repair and turnover, in addition to less water for cellular reactions involved in the countless metabolic reactions which occur in the cells. Thus, chronic dehydration can contribute to breakdown of the musculoskeletal system over time.

In regard to the intervertebral discs of the spine, they are known to have no blood supply and receive nutrients and oxygen by the capillaries from the vertebral bodies above and below. Smoking one cigarette is known to decrease the blood flow to the discs by 50% within one minute of smoking the cigarette. Dehydration similarly decreases the capillary pressure and thus accelerates degeneration of the discs.

In regard to headaches, if we are dehydrated, we may not have enough reserve water to produce the 600-700 ml (20-23 ounces) of cerebrospinal fluid that the body produces daily to protect and nourish the spinal cord and brain. If we are dehydrated, we may develop a positional or dehydration headache. The brain is made up of approximately 85% water. If we are dehydrated, the dehydrated brain can temporarily contract or shrink from fluid loss. This causes the brain to pull away from the skull causing pain and resulting in a dehydration headache that can range from mild to as severe and debilitating as a migraine. Rehydration will rapidly rehydrate the brain and reverse the process and the pain.

Most of us (including me), find it difficult to drink the recommended amount of water (8-10 eight-ounce glasses per day for individuals who do not have heart or kidney failure). This is because we either don't have time to stop and drink water or we don't have time to go to the bathroom due to our frenetic nonstop schedules. Since coffee, tea, alcohol, and sugar-containing drinks are actually dehydrating, these do not count as rehydrating your body. If you are an athlete or work at a very physical job, you may need to replace the water your body loses during the course of your activity. If we are rapidly hydrating or hydrating over the course of the day with more than one half to two liters of water, we should make sure we are adding a small amount (one half teaspoon) of salt to our water or drinking coconut water or electrolyte-containing water.

Finally, it is most important to focus on a complete and balanced nutritional program, with emphasis on whole natural food sources when possible (since there are many co-factors and other chemicals found naturally in food which help to optimally assimilate various nutrients and prevent harmful effects). Focus on a balanced diet that doesn't leave anything major out or leave you very low in any important nutrient. There is no one magic bullet. The body needs all the essential components, including the emotional and mental state that contributes to optimal digestion and assimilation of nutrients, in order to function well and be healthy and to heal chronic pain and disease. In addition, we are all unique, amazingly and beautifully different, necessary and complementary to each other in regard to culture, beliefs, and individual tastes. There are healthy substitutes for many traditional dishes. Do your own research and enjoy this process.

Enjoy creating your own blue zone filled with the rich colorful, textured healthy diet, loving healthy supportive and sustaining human connections, activities which you love which move and strengthen your body, and rituals of mindfulness which transform and rebuild you. I wish you a deeply meaningful and transformative journey of healing and wellbeing.

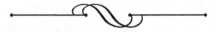

Exercise/meditation: seeing your life

Sit in a quiet place where you will not be disturbed. If necessary, support your back with pillows so that you are sitting comfortably with your back and neck in a neutral position, feet flat on the floor in front of you, hands resting on your thighs. Observe your breathing, relax and slow your breathing. Allow your abdomen to naturally expand with your in-breath and fall back without effort with your exhale. When you are ready, travel or be transported to your healing place or sanctuary. You can modify it in any way that improves your feeling of contentment and well-being. Pay attention to each area of your body, your thoughts, and emotions which need healing with compassion and send them thoughts and support for healing. In this safe place, allow yourself to see yourself in your ideal environment, location(s), work, friends, and situations as if you had the ability to create your ideal life. Imagine activities and the type of movement and exercise that you would ideally enjoy. Visualize yourself fit, healthy, vibrant, doing the things you love to do, eating your ideal beautifully prepared, delicious, healthy foods.

Now look back at your life, as if you were standing at the end and looking back. Ask yourself what you would have said, done, dared, and accomplished that you were afraid to do, did not dare to do, did not try to do because of fear, anger, or convention. Now ask yourself what you are most grateful for in the life that you have lived. What have you done or accomplished which left you breathless, which took courage, strength, grace, or integrity? Now, relax and observe your breath. Think of one thing which you can do now to create the life that you want to live … a life of health and well-being, joy and connection, a live filled with meaningful moments, cherished daily rituals, new beginnings, and gratitude. Ask for guidance from your unconscious self, from the source of life, the source of breath. You can come back to this place and exercise at any time. Now, when you feel that you are satisfied for today, slowly travel back to the current time and place and open your eyes.

Conclusion:

CREATING A NEW PARADIGM FOR HEALTH AND MEDICINE

"An ounce of prevention is worth a pound of cure"
– Benjamin Franklin

Although "We the People" are the founding power of the great democracy that is the United States of America, we often forget the ability that we have as individuals, groups, and consumers to change the current approach to medical care, to advocate for educational and preventive approaches. According to Mathew Fenwick from the American Hospital Association on September 7, 2011, "Hospitals across the nation are responding to patient demand and integrating complementary and alternative medicine (CAM) services with the conventional services they normally provide, according to the results of a new survey released by Health Forum, a subsidiary of the American Hospital Association (AHA) and Samueli Institute, a non-profit research organization that investigates healing oriented practices. The survey shows that more than 42 percent of responding hospitals indicated they offer one or more CAM therapies, up from 37 percent in 2007." (1)

I believe that we can reverse the opioid crises through early education, public health education programs, and preventive strategies. We can reduce the transition of acute to chronic pain through early education and preventive strategies for mental and physical health. We can educate children, parents, young adults, and the elderly on the risk factors associated with the development of chronic pain and how to attain self-efficacy. I believe that as citizens, community members, employees, and owners of businesses and corporations, we have the potential to recoup the enormous human potential and financial resources which are now lost to the costs of chronic pain, suffering, and disability.

Although more physicians and allied health professionals are being trained in the fields of Integrative Medicine, Functional Medicine, and a holistic wellness approach to medicine, it is the medical consumer who is driving the demand for these services. Dr. David Eisenberg reported in his landmark article published in *The Journal of the American Medical Association* in 1998 that in 1997 visits to CAM practitioners exceeded visits to primary care physicians by more than 243 million. He reported that consumers were looking for natural therapies, healthy diets, and information regarding the benefit of nutrition, exercise, and stress reduction strategies to prevent disease with less focus on the diagnosis and treatment of symptoms and chronic disease. (2)

In 2015, the United States spent almost three times as much on healthcare on average compared to other countries with comparable incomes, according to data from the Organization for Economic Cooperation and Development. "The U.S. spends more money, but we definitely have worse health outcomes," said David Squires, president of the Commonwealth Fund, a private foundation based in New York that carries out independent research on healthcare issues. Despite investing heavily in healthcare, Americans live shorter lives than people in 30 other countries, data from the World Health Organization showed. In 2013, more people died in the United States from preventable diseases or complications than those in twelve other high-income countries, according to data from the European Observatory on Health Systems and Policies, a health policy organization with offices around Europe. (3)

According to the World Health Organization, the number one cause of death in developed nations is now chronic preventable disease, although we have the science and the knowledge to significantly decrease the risk for and occurrence of chronic disease. (4)

Advances in public health services during the 20th century including availability of clean food and water supplies, vaccines, and workplace safety regulations have resulted in an increase of the average lifespan in the United States of more than thirty years (all races, male, female combined). However, due to the highly processed and energy-dense modern diet, high levels of stress, and sedentary lifestyles, large numbers of individuals now surviving to middle and old age suffer from chronic disease which has been shown to be largely preventable and treatable with changes in behavior and lifestyle. (5)

Health economists from Johns Hopkins University writing in *The Journal of Pain* reported the annual cost of chronic pain is as high as $635 billion a year, which is more than the combined yearly costs for cancer, heart disease, and diabetes.

The authors noted their conclusions are conservative because the analysis did not consider the costs of pain for institutionalized and non-civilian populations, for persons under eighteen and for caregivers (Darrell J. Gaskin, Patrick Richard). (6)

I remember talking to an orthopedic surgeon colleague of mine about the preventive approach used by Pittsburg orthopedic surgeon Dr. Vonda Wright, author of *Fitness after 40: How to Stay Strong at Any Age,* who works with middle age and senior athletes and teaches them how to become active while reducing the risk of injury. He made the comment (tongue in cheek, yet very honest in regard to our current focus on treatment versus prevention), that if he focused on preventing injury, he would not have as many people to operate on.

Instead of believing in a scarcity model, I believe that visionary corporations, health insurance companies, and hospital systems can use American ingenuity and perseverance to create an economic model that creates increased national financial health and growth as it focuses on health, preventive approaches and well-being, which have the potential to recapture the lost productivity of the discouraged and disabled.

The most profitable and successful businesses and corporations invest in their workforce, in addition to their product, emphasizing long term well-being, creativity, and loyalty which increase productivity as a natural byproduct. If indeed, as described by renowned Physicist Frijof Capra and biologist Bruce Lipton, our society is its own ecosystem, a living system, then the health and well-being of our society as a whole, depends on how we value the most vulnerable among us.

ACKNOWLEDGEMENTS

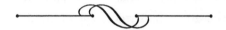

I could not have written this book without the encouragement of my many patients whose courage and commitment to healing from pain is a continuous inspiration to me and drives me to always be at my best and to always improve for their sake. I am also grateful to my dear family and friends for their support, wisdom, encouragement, humor, and comfort during times of suffering in my life. Thank you for encouraging me to make this information more available to patients suffering from chronic pain.

I owe much of the essential content of this book to the many scientists and authors whose work I have quoted in this book. They have each devoted their lives to advancing the science of human well-being and potential. These include Dr. Andrew Weil, who has had a great influence on my view of health, well-being, and the preventive, integrative and holistic approach to patient care at a critical time in my medical education. From that time until now, he has continued to be a leader in advancing the field of integrative medicine. I must acknowledge the other leaders, scientists, and leaders in this field whose work I have referenced: Dr. Dean Ornish, Dr. Larry Dossey, Physicists Frijof Capra and Carlo Rovelli, Dr. Herbert Benson and

Dr. Jon Cabot Zen, Dr. Candace Pert, Dr. Norman Doidge, Dr. Michael Moskowitz and Dr. Marla Golden, and the many other authors and scientists whose tireless dedication and work continues to contribute to our understanding of reality, living systems, health, healing, and well-being.

I am grateful to Dr. Joseph Helms of the Helms Medical Institute and his team of brilliant and dedicated instructors who are giants upon whose shoulders I stand when utilizing holistic Eastern medicine approaches to aid in harmonizing of mind, body, and spirit. I am forever grateful to Master Jiro Murai and Mary Burmeister for their exceptional lifelong dedication to researching, discovering, teaching, and living the ancient healing art of Jin Shin Jyutsu and for the international instructors who have continued to bring the understanding of how to simply "be" and know that all that we need to heal is within oneself, to countless people throughout the world.

I would like to acknowledge my many dedicated professors and teachers throughout my undergraduate education at Northern Arizona University. Their doors were always open and their curiosity and dedication to the search for solutions and knowledge and understanding was infectious. I caught the bug!

I will always be grateful to my older brother, mentor, and example, Dr. John Hunt. His courage in overcoming many daunting life challenges in addition to his tireless dedication to serving the very often abandoned and neglected patient with the dual diagnosis of chronic pain and addiction has inspired me to always see the person and not just the disease.

I would like to acknowledge my professors at the University of Arizona where I look back and see that I was privileged to have the most innovative and cutting edge medical education imaginable. I am grateful to all of my classmates in medical school who filled the years of learning with laughter and collegiality and with whom I traveled the exciting and demanding journey of becoming a physician.

I am grateful to the many physicians and faculty who mentored and taught me tirelessly during long days and nights on the wards, in the clinics, and in the operating room during my internship and residency at Naval Medical Center San Diego. It would take an entire book to list all of the enlisted staff, officers, colleagues, physicians, nurses, physical therapists, psychologists, pharmacists, corpsmen, government service and contractor staff with whom I have been privileged to work during my twenty-eight years as an active duty physician and Officer of the United States Navy. Now as a contractor, I am honored to be able to continue to work with these dedicated and selfless physicians and allied health care providers. They have tirelessly and happily devoted their lives to serving and caring for the men and women of the armed services. I am privileged to be associated with such honorable physicians, nurses, and medical team members whose lives are predicated upon providing the best of medical care to each patient, who treat each service member, retired service member, and their families as if they were their own beloved family members. I would like to mention with deep gratitude Captain John Dekrey, Captain Thomas Scanlan, Captain Jerry Berger, Captain David Leivers, Captain Bruce Laverty, Captain John Shapira, and Captain Gregory Gullahorn whose memories and influence are engraved in the hearts and minds of all who had the privilege to be trained under their watch and tutelage and our current Department Chair, Commander Scott Wallace, who is carrying on the tradition of excellence in service to the service members and their families who we are dedicated to care for. I will always be grateful to the mentorship, consummate example, and friendship of Captain Art Kelleher, Captain Brian Wamsley, Captain Ken Wingler, Captain Patrick Danaher, and Commander Kathleen MacDonald.

I also will be forever grateful to the "heart of the Pain Clinic" at Naval Medical Center San Diego, Rosa Owen RN Rose, after a lifetime of longer-than-expected days where you would not leave without meeting each patient's needs. You are finally able to spend time fly-fishing with Pat and being in your garden. Lam Yuet, pain service pharmacist extraordinaire, thank you for your friendship and your key role across the years in helping us to care for our patients. Hope to visit you in Hong Kong soon. Thank you to my dear friends in Okinawa and here in the United States for your encouragement and for the connection of spirit and joy of the journey of life that bridges the continent and the world.

I was so very privileged to undergo fellowship training at the Arnold-Warfield Pain Clinic at Beth Israel Deaconess Hospital in Boston. I will forever remember and be grateful for the knowledge and example of true physicians and healers imparted to me by Dr. Zahid Bajwa, Dr. Joshua Wooton, Dr. Thomas Simopolis, Dr. Joystna Nagda, Dr. Christine Peters Asdourian, and many others to whom I will always be in debt for their tireless dedication to mentoring and training future generations of physicians dedicated to the treatment of patients who suffer from chronic pain.

Thank you, Norman Plotkin at Author Incubator. You gave me the support and courage to say yes to the challenge and to begin what seemed to be such a daunting task. Thank you, Angela Lauria, for making Difference Press a reality and for encouraging and supporting the dream of those of us looking to make a difference in the lives of others. Thank you, Cheyenne, for checking in and encouraging me along the way. That meant more than you know. I am so grateful also to my editor Bethany for her inspired guidance, which has helped to make the technical aspects of this book more accessible to my patients and readers, to Author Incubator Production Coordinator

Chela Hardy for her invaluable assistance, and to all of editors and staff of Difference Press who helped make this book a reality.

To the Morgan James Publishing team: Special thanks to David Hancock, CEO & Founder for believing in me and my message. To my Author Relations Manager, Bonnie Rauch, thank you for your expertise which made the process seamless and simple, which was so essential to the complex balancing act of my life. Many more thanks to everyone else, but especially Jim Howard, Bethany Marshall, and Nickcole Watkins.

I am forever grateful to my husband and best friend of twenty-four years, Stephen. Thank you for your belief in me, for loving me as I am, for being such a wonderful father, for always making me laugh and for your endless patience with the years of long days and nights away while taking care of my patients. I am grateful to my parents, Jay Byron Hunt, PhD and my mother Roberta Elizabeth Macknight Hunt. You showed me that success is based on persistence and on getting back up no matter how many times you fall down. Thank you for imparting to me your love of learning, your love of work, your love of people, and your love of service to others. Thank you to our precious Ethan for saving my life … for giving me a second chance at life. You are our hero. We were blessed and honored by each moment and day you were here with us and I know that you are with us still in spirit. I owe an incalculable debt to Dr. Brian Auge and Dr. James L'Esperance for your consummate skill as surgeons and physicians and your humanity, which also saved my life. Finally, thank you Vera, Kathleen and Kristine for friendships of a lifetime.

THANK YOU

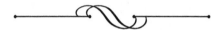

Thank you for reading *Pain Is Not What It Seems*. If you have come to this page, it is a sign that you have not given up. Thank you for your courage, your hope, your strength, and your will to transform a life of suffering and pain into one of meaning, inner peace, and joy.

I know, from many decades of caring for patients with chronic pain, that you are someone who has taken on monumental life challenges to the point of finally breaking down.

Thank you for taking this journey with me to the beginning of a new odyssey, a deeper discovery of the extraordinary and unique human being that you are and the rare gifts that only you can share with others during this lifelong journey into healing.

If you are interested in working with others to transform healthcare, education, your home, and the workplace into environments that promote prevention, health, and well-being, please message me on LinkedIn for a list of next steps.

https://www.linkedin.com/in/anita-hickey-74680233/

ABOUT THE AUTHOR

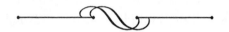

D r. Hickey completed a Bachelor of Science degree in chemistry from Northern Arizona University *summa cum laude* prior to attending medical school at University of Arizona. She completed her transitional internship and residency in anesthesiology at Naval Medical Center San Diego and a

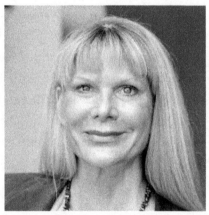

(Apr 19, 1953 – Feb 19, 2019)

post-doctoral fellowship in pain management at the Arnold-Warfield Pain Management Center at Harvard's Beth Israel Deaconess Medical Center and Children's Hospital in Boston. She was board certified in Anesthesiology, Pain Management (ABA) and Integrative Medicine (ABIHM). As Senior Navy Medical acupuncturist, she mentored more than 150 medical acupuncturists.

Dr. Hickey served in many leadership positions, authored numerous peer-reviewed publications and book chapters on topics including pain management, Stellate Ganglion Block for post-traumatic stress disorder, and acupuncture. She spoke at numerous medical conferences on Integrative Medicine and Pain Management. In addition, she participated in numerous working groups on pain management and integrative medicine for the Department of Defense and the VA. She was selected as the Integrative Medicine and Pain Medicine United States Navy representative for the Army Surgeon General's task force on pain management, whose report recommending a holistic, multidisciplinary, and multimodal pain management strategy was published in 2010. She was awarded multiple honors and awards, including the Meritorious Service Medal, Navy and Marine Corps Commendation Medal with two stars, Navy Meritorious Unit Medal, Humanitarian Service Medal with star, Overseas Medal with Star, Sea Service Medal, NATO Medal, South East Asia Medal, and Navy Expeditionary Medal.

Dr. Hickey resided in San Diego, California with her husband, daughter and their cat, Queen Elizabeth.

REFERENCES

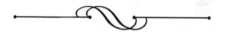

Introduction:

1. U.S. Department of Veterans Affairs. Whole Health For Life: Expanding the VA Whole Health System. https://www.va.gov/PATIENTCENTEREDCARE/features/Expanding_the_VA_Whole_Health_System.asp.

2. Eisenberg, David M., R. B. Davis, S. L. Ettner, S. Appel, S. Wilkey, M. Van Rompay, and R. C. Kessler. "Trends in Alternative Medicine Use in the United States, 1990-1997: Results of a Follow-up National Survey." *JAMA* 280, no. 18 (November 11, 1998): 1569-575. Accessed May 10, 2018. https://jamanetwork.com/journals/jama/fullarticle/188148.

Chapter 2:

1. International Association for the Study of Pain. Acute Pain. Accessed May 10, 2018. https://www.iasp-pain.org/TaxonomyTransition from acute to chronic pain

2. Li, Qian-Qian, Guang-Xia Shi, Cun-Zhi Liu, and Lin-Peng Wang. "Acupuncture Effect and Central Autonomic Regulation." *Evidence-Based Complementary and Alternative*

*Medicine*2013 (2013). Accessed May 10, 2018. http://dx.doi.org/10.1155/2013/267959.

3. Ferzerfan, A., and G. Sheh. "Transition from Acute to Chronic Pain." *Continuing Education in Anaesthesia Critical Care & Pain* 15, no. 2 (April 1, 2015): 98-102. Accessed May 10, 2018. https://doi.org/10.1093/bjaceaccp/mku044.

4. Sharar, S. R., W. Miller, A. Teeley, M. Soltani, H. G. Hoffman, M. P. Jensen, and D. R. Patterson. "Applications of Virtual Reality for Pain Management in Burn-injured Patients." *Expert Review of Neurotherapeutics* 8, no. 11 (November 2008): 1667-674. Accessed May 10, 2018. https://dx.doi.org/10.1586/14737175.8.11.1667.

5. Chapman, C. R., R. P. Tuckett, and C. W. Song. "Pain and Stress in a Systems Perspective: Reciprocal Neural, Endocrine, and Immune Interactions." *The Journal of Pain* 9, no. 2 (February 2008): 122-45. Accessed May 10, 2018. https://www.ncbi.nlm.nih.gov/pmc/articles/PMC2278005/.

6. Lazar, Sara W., Catherine E. Kerr, Rachehel H. Wasserman, Jeremy R. Gray, Douglas N. Greeve, Michael T. Treadway, Metta Mcgarvey, Brian T. Quinn, Jeffrey A. Dusek, Herbert Bensen, Scott L. Rauch, Christopher I. Moore, and Bruce Fischl. "Meditation Experience Is Associated with Increased Cortical Thickness." *Neuroreport* 16, no. 17 (November 28, 2005): 1893-897. Accessed May 10, 2018. https://www.ncbi.nlm.nih.gov/pmc/articles/PMC1361002/#__ffn_sectitle.

7. Ornish, Dean. *The Spectrum: How to Customize a Way of Eating and Living Just Right for You and Your Family.* New York, NY: Ballentine Books, 2008.

8. Brownstein, Arthur H. *Healing Back Pain Naturally: The Mind-Body Program Proven to Work.* New York, NY: Pocket Books, 2001.

9. Moskowitz, Michael, and Marla Golden. Neuroplastix: Change the Brain; Relieve the Pain; Transform the Person. 2015. Accessed May 10, 2018. http://www.neuroplastix.com.

10. Doige, Norman. *The Brain's Way of Healing: Remarkable Discoveries and Recoveries from the Frontiers of Neuroplasticity.* New York, NY: Penguin Books, 2015, 2016.

11. Doige, Norman. *The Brain That Changes Itself: Stories of Triumph from the Frontiers of Brain Science.* New York, NY: Penguin Books, 2007.

12. Capra, Fritjof, and Pier Luigi Luisi. *The System's View of Life: A Unifying Vision.* New York, NY: Cambridge University Press, 2014.

I highly recommend this book. It is a product of 30 years of discussion with the most brilliant scientists of our time that helps us to understand the background, current understanding and scientific conception of life in regard to medicine and health, politics, economics and psychology.

Chapter 3:

1. Pert, Candace B., M. R. Ruff, R. J. Weber, and M. Herkenham. "Neuropeptides and Their Receptors: A Psychosomatic Network." *Journal of Immunology* 135, no. 2 (August 1, 1985): 820-26. Accessed May 10, 2018. http://www.jimmunol.org/content/135/2/820.

2. Hasenbring, M., D. Hallner, and B. Klasen. "Psychological Mechanisms in the Transition from Acute to Chronic Pain: Over or Underrated?" *Schmerz* 15, no. 6 (December 2001): 442-47. doi:https://doi.org/10.1007/s004820100030.

3. Pincus, T., A. K. Burton, S. Vogel, and A. P. Field. "A Systematic Review of Psychological Factors as Predictors of Chronicity/ disability in Prospective Cohorts of Low Back Pain." *Spine*

27, no. 5 (March 1, 2002): E109-120. Accessed May 10, 2018. https://www.ncbi.nlm.nih.gov/pubmed/11880847.

4. Frentzel-Beyme, R., and R. Grossarth-Maticek. "The Interaction between Risk Factors and Self-regulation in the Development of Chronic Diseases." *International Journal of Hygiene and Environmental Health* 204, no. 1 (October 2001): 81-88. Accessed May 10, 2018. doi:DOI: 10.1078/1438-4639-00077.

5. Morasco, Benjamin J., Bobbi Jo Yarborough, Ning X. Smith, Steven K. Dobscha, Richard A. Deyo, Nancy A. Perrin, and Carla A. Green. ". Higher Prescriptions Opioid Dose Is Associated with Worse Patient-reported Pain Outcomes and More Health Care Utilization." *The Journal of Pain* 18, no. 4 (April 2017): 437-45. Accessed May 10, 2018. doi:https://doi.org/10.1016/j.jpain.2016.12.004.

6. Tick, Heather. "Integrative Pain Medicine: A Holistic Model of Care." International Association for the Study of Pain IASP: Pain, Clinical Update. May 2014. Accessed May 10, 2018. http://americanpainsociety.org/uploads/get-involved/iasp-clinical-update.pdf.

7. Institute of Medicine 2011 report: "Relieving Pain in America: Blueprint for Transforming Prevention, Care, Education and Research. Accessed May 10, 2018 https://www.ncbi.nlm.nih.gov/books/NBK91497/pdf/Bookshelf_NBK91497.pdf

8. Rein, Glen, Mike Atkinson, and Rollin McCraty. "The Physiological and Psychological Effects of Compassion and Anger." *Journal of Advancement in Medicine* 8, no. 2 (Summer 1995): 87-105. Accessed May 10, 2018. https://www.heartmath.org/assets/uploads/2015/01/compassion-and-anger.pdf.

9. McCraty, Rollin, Bob Barrios-Choplin, Deborah Rozman, Mike Atkinson, and Alan D. Watkins. "The Impact of a New Emotional Self-Management Program on Stress, Emotions, Heart Rate Variability, DHEA and Cortisol. Police Officers: In Search of Coherence and Resilience." *Integrative Physiological and Behavioral Science* 33, no. 2 (Spring 1998): 151-70. Accessed May 10, 2018. https://www.heartmath. org/assets/uploads/2015/01/dhea-cortisol-study.pdf.

10. https://www.connectthemind.com/blog/2017/12/6/freeze-frame-technique-from-heart-math-institute

Chapter 4:

1. 1.Benson, Herbert. *Timeless Healing: The Power and Biology of Belief.* New York, NY: Simon and Shuster, 1997. page 30

2. Beecher, Henry K. "The Powerful Placebo." *JAMA* 159, no. 17 (1955): 1602-606.AccessedMay17,2018. doi:doi:10.1001/jama.1955.02960340022006.

3. 3.Moerman, Daniel E., and Wayne B. Jonas. "Deconstructing the Placebo Effect and Finding the Meaning Response." *Annals of Internal Medicine* 136 (March 19, 2002): 471-76. Accessed May 10, 2018. yqy http://annals.org/aim/article-abstract/715182/deconstructing-placebo-effect-finding-meaning-response? volume=136&issue=6&page=471.

4. Egbert, Lawrence D., George E. Battit, Claude E. Welch, and Marshall K. Bartlett. "Reduction of Postoperative Pain by Encouragement and Instruction of Patients. A Study of Doctor-Patient Rapport." *New England Journal of Medicine* 270, no. 16 (1964): 825-27. Accessed May 10, 2018. doi: https://www.nejm.org/doi/full/10.1056/NEJM196404162701606.

5. Chapin, Heather, E. Bagarinao, and S. Mackey. "Real-time FMRI Applied to Pain Management." Neuroscience Letters

520, no. 2 (June 29, 2012): 174-81. Accessed May 10, 2018. https://www.ncbi.nlm.nih.gov/pmc/articles/PMC3377818/.

Chapter 5:

1. Chodren, Pema. "How to Practice Tonglin". The Lion's Roar: Buddhist Wisdom for Our Time. November 9, 2017. Accessed 11 May 2018.. https://www.lionsroar.com/how-to-practice-tonglen/

2. *Pema Chodron and Alice Walker in Conversation on the Meaning of Suffering and the Mystery of Joy.* Directed by Alice Walker, Pema Chodron. Louisville, Colorado. Sounds True Publishing. 1999. DVD.

3. *Fail, Fail Again, Fail Better. Wise advise for Leaning into the Unknown.* Directed by Pema Chodron. Loisville Colorado. Sounds True Publishing. 2015. E-book.

4. Lown, Bernard. *The Lost Art of Healing: Practicing Compassion in Medicine.* New York, NY: Ballantine Books, 1996, 1999.

Chapter 6:

1. Kim, Dae-Keun, Jyoo-HI Rhee, and Seung Wan Kang. "Reorganization of the Brain and Heart Rhythm during Autogenic Meditation." *Frontiers in Integrative Neuroscience* 7 (January 13, 2014): 1-9. Accessed May 11, 2018. doi:doi: 10.3389/fnint.2013.00109, article 109

2. Tyagi, Anupama, and Marc Cohen. "Yoga and Heart Rate Variability: A Comprehensive Review of the Literature." *International Journal of Yoga* 9, no. 2 (July 2016): 97-113. Accessed May 11, 2018. https://www.ncbi.nlm.nih.gov/pmc/articles/PMC4959333/.

3. Burmeister, Mary. *1. Text 2: Physio-Philosophy,(Nature Effortless Reality): Jin Shin Jyutsu·: Cosmic Artless Art to Know (Help) Myself.*

Page 14 Scottsdale, AZ: Jin Shin Jyutsu, 1992. A Mary Burmeister; and JSJinc.net website. Link *About Mary*. https://www.jsjinc.net/pagedetails.php? id=about-mary referenced 3/29/2018

4. Malenbaum, Sara, Francis J. Keefe, Amanda Williams, Roger Ulrich, and Tamara J. Somers. "Pain in Its Environmental Context: Implications for Designing Environments to Enhance Pain Control." *Pain* 134, no. 3 (February 2008): 241-44. Accessed May 11, 2018. https://www.ncbi.nlm.nih.gov/pmc/articles/PMC2264925/pdf/nihms-38645.pdf.

Chapter 7:

1. Tonosu, Juichi, Hirjoyuki Oka, Ko Matsudaira, Akiro Higashikawa, Hiroshi Okazaki, and Sakae Tanaka. "The Relationship between Findings on Magnetic Resonance Imaging and Previous History of Low Back Pain." *Journal of Pain Research* 10 (December 29, 2016): 47-52. Accessed May 11, 2018. https://www.ncbi.nlm.nih.gov/pmc/articles/PMC5214701/pdf/jpr-10-047.pdf.

2. Tonosu, Juichi, Akiro Higashikawa, Hiroshi Okasaki, Sakae Tanaka, and Ko Matsadiaira. "The Associations between Magnetic Resonance Imaging Findings and Low Back Pain: A 10-year Longitudinal Analysis." *PLoS ONE*12, no. 11 (November 15, 2017). Accessed May 11, 2018. doi: https://doi.org/10.1371/journal.pone.0188057.

3. Bohman, Tony, Lars Alfredsson, Irene Jensen, Johan Hallqvist, Eva Vingard, and Eva Stillgate. "Does a Healthy Lifestyle Behavior Influence the Prognosis of Low Back Pain among Men and Women in a General Population? A Populagion-based Cohor Study." *BMJ Open* 4, no. 12 (December 30, 2014). Accessed May 11, 2018. http://bmjopen.bmj.com/content/4/12/e005713.

Chapter 8:

1. Gezen-ak, Duygu, Erdinç Dursun, and Selma Yilmazer "The Effect of Vitamin D Treatment on Nerve Growth Factor Release from Hippocampal Neurons." *NoroPsikiyatri* 51, no. 2 (June 2014): 157-62. Accessed May 12, 2018. https://www.ncbi.nlm.nih.gov/pmc/articles/PMC5353091/.

2. Malloy, Peter J., and David Feldman. "Genetic Disorders and Defects in Vitamin D Action." *Endocrinology and Metabolism Clinics of North America* 39, no. 2 (June 2010): 333-46. Accessed May 12, 2018. https://www.ncbi.nlm.nih.gov/pmc/articles/PMC2879401/.

3. Hollis, Bruce W., and Carol L. Wagner. "Vitamin D and Pregnancy: Skeletal Effects, Non-skeletal Effects and Birth Outcomes." *Calcified Tissue International* 92, no. 2 (February 2013): 128-39. Accessed May 12, 2018. https://link.springer.com/article/10.1007/s00223-012-9607-4.

4. National Institute of Health Office of Dietary Supplements. "Vitamin D: Factsheet for Health Professionals." National Institute of Health Office of Dietary Supplements. March 2, 2018. Accessed May 12, 2018. https://ods.od.nih.gov/factsheets/VitaminD-HealthProfessional/.

5. Hollick, Michael F., Neil C. Binckley, Heike A. Bischoff-Ferrari, Catherine M. Gordon, David A. Hanley, Robert P. Heaney, M. Hassan Murad, and Connie M. Weaver. "Evaluation, Treatment and Prevention of Vitamin D Deficiency: An Endocrine Society Clinical Practice Guideline." *The Journal of Clinical Endocrinology & Metabolism* 96, no. 7 (June 6, 2011): 1911-930. Accessed May 12, 2018. https://doi.org/10.1210/jc.2011-0385.

6. Wagner, Carol L., Rebecca McNeil, and Bruce W. Hollis. "A Randomized Trial of Vitamin D Supplementation in Two

Community Health Center Networks in South Carolina." *American Journal of Obstetrics and Gynecology* 208, no. 2 (February 2013): 137.el-37.13. Accessed May 12, 2018. https://www.ncbi.nlm.nih.gov/pmc/articles/PMC4365423/.

7. "Dietary Guidelines For Americans 2015-20120 Eighth Edition." Health.gov. December 2015. Accessed May 12, 2018. https://health.gov/dietaryguidelines/2015/resources/2015-2020 Dietary Guidelines.pdf.

8. Wei, Min, Sebastian Brandhorst, Mahshid Shelehchi, Hamed Mirzaei, Chia Weng Cheng, Julia Budniak, Susan Groshen, Wendy J. Mack, Esra Guen, Stefano Di Biase, Pinchas Cohen, Todd E. Morgan, Tanya Dorff, Kurt Hong, Andreas Michalsen, Alessandro Laviano, and Valter D. Longo. "Fasting-mimicking Diet and Markers/risk Factors for Aging, Diabetes, Cancer and Cardiovascular Disease." *Science Translational Medicine* 9, no. 377 (February 15, 2017): Eaai8700. Accessed May 12, 2018. doi:DOI: 10.1126/scitranslmed.aai8700.

9. Brandhorst, S., and V. D. Longo. "Fasting and Caloric Restriction in Cancer Prevention and Treatment." *Recent Results Cancer Research* 207 (2016): 241-66. Accessed May 12, 2018. doi:doi: 10.1007/978-3-319-42118-6_12.

10. Weil, Andrew. *Fast Food, Good Food: More Than 150 Quick and Easy Ways to Put Healthy, Delicious Food on the Table.* New York, NY: Little Brown and Company, 2015.

11. Barcizewski, Jan, Janusz Jurczak, Sylwester Porowski, Thomas Specht, and Volker A. Erdmann. "The Role of Water in Conformational Changes of Nucleic Acids in Ambient and High Pressure Conditions." *European Journal of Biochemistry* 260 (December 25, 2001): 293-07. Accessed May 12, 2018. doi: https://doi.org/10.1046/j.1432-1327.1999.00184.x.

Conclusion:

1. Fenwick, Matthew, and David Hutcheson. "More Hospitals Offering Complementary and Alternative Medicine Services." American Hospital Association. September 7, 2011. Accessed May 12, 2018. https://www.aha.org/system/files/presscenter/pressrel/2011/110907-pr-camsurvey.pdf.

2. Eisenberg, David M., R. B. Davis, S. L. Ettner, S. Appel, S. Wilkey, M. Van Rompay, and R. C. Kessler. "Trends in Alternative Medicine Use in the United States, 1990-1997: Results of a Follow-up National Survey." *JAMA*280, no. 18 (November 11, 1998): 1569-575. Accessed May 10, 2018. https://jamanetwork.com/journals/jama/fullarticle/188148.

3. Etehad, Melissa, and Kyle Kim. "The U.S. Spends More on Healthcare than Any Other Country – but Not with Better Health Outcomes." *Los Angeles Times*, July 18, 2017. Accessed May 13, 2018. http://www.latimes.com/nation/la-na-healthcare-comparison-20170715-htmlstory.html.

4. World Health Organization. "Integrated Chronic Disease Prevention and Control." Chronic Diseases and Health Promotion. 2018. Accessed May 13, 2018. http://www.who.int/chp/about/integrated_cd/en/.

5. Centers for Disease Control and Prevention. "Ten Great Public Health Achievements – United States, 1900-1999" *Morbidity and Mortality Weekly Report.*48, no. 12 (April 2,1999):241-243. Accessed May 13, 2018. https://www.cdc.gov/mmwr/preview/mmwrhtml/00056796.htm

6. Gaskin, D. J., and P. Richard. "The Economic Costs of Pain in the United States." *The Journal of Pain* 13, no. 8 (August 2012): 715-24. doi:doi: 10.1016/j.jpain.2012.03.009.

NOTES

Printed in the USA
CPSIA information can be obtained
at www.ICGtesting.com
JSHW081545291123
52955JS00005B/310

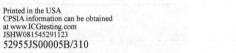

9 781642 793000